AFTER
AUSCHWITZ:
A LOVE STORY

Other books by Brenda Webster:

Fiction:

Vienna Triangle

The Beheading Game

Sins of the Mothers

Paradise Farm

Drama:

The Murder Trial of Sigmund Freud (with Meridee Stein)

Memoir:

The Last Good Freudian

Translation:

Lettera alla Madre, by Edith Bruck

Critical Studies:

Yeats: A Psychoanalytic Study

Blake's Prophetic Psychology

Edited:

Hungry for Light: The Journal of Ethel Schwabacher

AFTER AUSCHWITZ: A LOVE STORY

Brenda Webster

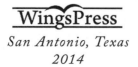

WingsPress

San Antonio, Texas
2014

After Auschwitz: A Love Story
© 2014 by Wings Press, for Brenda Webster

Cover image © 2013 by Guillermo Webster

First Edition

ISBN: 978-1-60940-359-1
paperback original

epub ISBN: 978-1-60940-360-7
Kindle ISBN: 978-1-60940-361-4
Library PDF ISBN: 978-1-60940-362-1

Wings Press
627 E. Guenther
San Antonio, Texas 78210
Phone/fax: (210) 271-7805
On-line catalogue and ordering: www.wingspress.com
All Wings Press titles are distributed to the trade by
Independent Publishers Group
www.ipgbook.com

Library of Congress Cataloging-in-Publication Data:

Webster, Brenda S.
  After Auschwitz : a love story / Brenda Webster.. -- First Edition.
    pages cm
  Includes index.
  ISBN 978-1-60940-359-1 (pbk. : alk. paper) -- ISBN 978-1-60940-360-7
(ePub ebook) -- ISBN 978-1-60940-361-4 (MobiPocket ebook) -- ISBN
978-1-60940-362-1 (pdf)
    1. Husband and wife--Fiction. 2. Diaries Authorship--Fiction. 3.
Alzheimer's disease--Fiction. 4. World War, 1939-1945 Prisoners and
prisons--Fiction. 5. Auschwitz (Concentration camp) Buildings--Fiction. 6.
Holocaust survivors--Fiction.
    I. Title.
  PS3573.E255 A69 2014
  813'.54   2013038604

Thanks to Lisa who designed the yellow lettering on the cover.
And special thanks to Rose Webster for her help
and to Sari Friedman for her caring and careful proofing.

To my husband, Ira,
and my children Lisa, Michael and Rebecca,
who are always there for me.
I couldn't have written this
without your support and love.

AFTER AUSCHWITZ: A LOVE STORY

Rome 2010

Hannah's brother Eddie used to dance with her when she was a child in their Romanian village, she told me, to make his wife jealous. Then, after the liberation of Auschwitz, when the war was over, Eddie pushed Hannah into an early marriage—so early it was ridiculous. She was only sixteen and had lived much of her short life in a death camp. Though she never admitted it, I got the feeling that she had been pregnant. Once Hannah was married, Eddie encouraged her to emigrate to Israel with him and their sister Leah. He painted a picture of the land of milk and honey. Instead, Hannah said, Israel became part of her nightmare. She and her boy-husband were housed in tin sheds, hot to the touch at midday, and after a week he was inducted into the army.

When she complained, Eddie and Leah were unsympathetic. Unlike Hannah, they had taken their dead mother's religion to Israel, clinging to it with ferocity. Naturally they expected Hannah to go along.

"I'm for peace," she'd tell them. "That means I hate the violence on either side." They shook their heads as if she were a *meshugeneh*.

I was impressed by the very things her family hated, Hannah's evocations of her Romanian village life: the sled made from an old platter, the river, the surrounding forest, and especially their poverty—poverty her siblings were ashamed of, just as they were ashamed of the brutal expulsion by their Christian neighbors. Hannah didn't deny the expulsion; she talked freely about it, admitted how it hurt her, even how it was the source of her phobias—her "stuckness" as she still calls it—but she also talked about running wild in the woods, getting mud all over her second-best dress, and being slapped by her mother when she came back because she played with the boys as though she had a right to some freedom.

In 1959, fourteen years after the liberation of the death camps, Eddie had a heart attack on the boat from Israel to Rome, where he was going to visit Hannah. While he was recovering, she tried to talk to him about their father's death. He wouldn't listen, couldn't talk about it. So instead she talked to me, lying with her head in my lap while I ran my fingers though her hair. I drew it out of her like a bee draining a flower.

I'll never forget the first time I saw her. She was chain-smoking, her blond plait down her back, thick and glossy. Her early marriage was over and she was surrounded by men. I say I'll never forget, but it's more accurate to say that it will be one of the last things to go when my memory is ultimately lost. I keep her photo in my pocket and take it out several times a day, communing.

It's easier to remember that Hannah than the one who sits at her typewriter, furiously typing day after day.

"Go away, Renzo," she says. "I'm working. Later we'll walk. I'll fix you a *spagettino*—you'll like that won't you? You go now, work a little on your poems. No, really, let me work for a bit! Weren't you the one always urging me to write?"

She has the slightest smile. I can't tell. There might even be a touch of malice.

"Be careful what you wish for," she says, smiling.

My poems are stillborn now. I lack the force to tie the isolated images together. Instead my thoughts flow easily to her at twenty with the blond braid and the blue eyes scanning my face, judging.

The year after she came to Rome there was a new documentary about the *Shoah* made by a friend of mine, a fellow director. I would gladly have gone alone but she insisted on coming too; she was always testing herself. Trying to comprehend the incomprehensible. Towards the end of the film, or maybe it was the beginning, there was an image of a pile of men—so thin that at first they seemed to be rags. It took a moment to make out the skeletal bones of hands or feet, bones barely covered with skin.

Suddenly, Hannah screamed and fell to the floor between the red velvet seats, tearing her hair. I dropped to my knees and put my arms around her, soothing her the way I would a heart-broken child. That night when we were lying in bed listening to the church chimes, she told me what had happened. Eddie and their father had been interned together. Eddie had gone out to work one day. When he got back their father wasn't in his bunk. Eddie finally found him in a pile of corpses. He said the prayer for the dead.

I held her while she cried. "I want to be close to you, Renzo," she mumbled, burrowing into my shoulder like a small animal. "But you've never even seen a dead person. You live here in a *palazzo* on top of the world and talk about death, about misery…you know nothing."

"A little," I said. "I know a little. My mother was very sick when I was small. If every minute you are awake you are afraid of dying, doesn't that… and my sister…"

"It's not the same," Hannah said.

"All right" I said. "I'm not going to argue about degrees of suffering." I caressed her back and murmured, comforting her. I knew even then that this wasn't a casual affair. I wanted to care for Hannah, protect her, heal her. She lived in a state of nightmare. I wanted to wake her up. I hadn't been able to do that for my mother, when I was a boy watching her pain.

The funny thing about my memory now is that I don't remember in straight lines with dates. Only flashes like stars in a black sky. I'm not even sure if before and after matter. But if I relax and let images come, it cheers me and makes me feel less alone.

The night was warm. We drank champagne and the crowd spilled out onto the street. Israel came up, as it often did, and someone, a woman, was defending the occupation of the West Bank as necessary. Hannah had had quite a bit to drink.

"You sound like a mother defending her child," she said, flushing. "The Shoah doesn't give us the right to mistreat the Arabs." She gave a bitter laugh. "But who am I to talk? My own family feels the way you do. They stare at me and roll their eyes as if I were mad. 'Give away Jerusalem? Never—we have it, let's keep it. The land is sacred.'"

She is stronger than she looks, this girl. She of all people might strike out blindly vengeful: half her family killed. Mother, father, brothers. But she is without the slightest sentimentality and rejects hatred.

"Jerusalem is an image of safety that everyone wants but only some people get," she says, her voice soft. I see the energy go out of her. Her walk slows, she leans on my arm, seems to get younger and younger as we walk home.

"Little one," I say holding her close, "Piccina." It is the same name I call her now even though I am the one who is weaker.

I started giving her baths one day when she'd been lying down with a bad headache. I thought it would relax her. She had so many physical symptoms left over from the camps.

What kind of a world do we have, where a twelve-year-old girl was made to drag corpses to a pit and throw them in?

Even the sound of the water was soothing, the steam, the fragrant bubbles making soft mounds in the tub—we were in our little bathroom, with its view of Borromini's cupola framed by sweet-smelling honeysuckle.

At first she resisted like a two-year-old wanting to do it herself, hands busy unbuttoning her blouse. I pushed her hands away.

"No," I told her, "Let me do it." I unzipped her skirt; it slipped down and fell to the tiled floor. I hung it on the brass hook next to her robe. Then I leaned over and tested the water.

"Perfect," I said looking at her breasts, nipples hardening under my gaze. Slowly, like a sleepwalker, one elegant leg at a time, she entered the bath. How I loved her body, the breasts voluptuous, and all the rest—waist, hips, thighs—still girlish.

Though I was older, you mustn't think that we were like father and child. Hannah was strongly sexual; or rather sex was one of the ways she ... by which she exerted her power. I think that in addition to wanting to help her and lull her, I felt I could possess her more thoroughly by bringing her back to childhood.

Looking at her, I wondered, not for the first time, whether she had been raped in the camps. But she said no. A young soldier had mocked her, spit on her, said that if she were a little older he would have taken her to bed, but no, no rape. I took the red washcloth off its peg and kneeling beside the tub, gently rubbed her back, her shoulders. She lifted her legs one after the other and I ran the cloth over them.

"Did your mother ever do this?" I asked.

She snorted. "I could never have imagined such a thing—with eight children to care for! Besides, we had no running water except what fell on us from the sky, dripping or pouring from the thatch of our hut. Sometimes we collected it in whatever bowl or tub came to hand or went down to the river with buckets. If it was winter we'd have to break through the ice."

"You sound angry. If it's at me, I'm sorry if I offended you."

"It's not you. It's not even the hut and its leaky thatch. It just reminds me of my mother—so infuriatingly accepting of everything. For instance, she always said it was impossible to feed so many mouths. Then one day I saw from her swollen belly that she was pregnant again. 'What?' I said, 'I thought we were too many already.'"

"'Shhh. It's God's will,' mother said. But I had grown up on the farm watching animals in rut. 'I thought you slept with

Papa,' I answered, and she slapped me across the mouth. So where was God that he didn't see how it was with us?"

Hannah sighed and slipped lower in the tub. I reached for the end of her blond plait, undid it and washed her hair, scratching her scalp, turning her head from side to side.

One of the cats slipped into the bathroom. The big black one—her favorite (she had five)—stood on its hind feet and peered into the tub, quizzical.

"I'll never have children," she told me soon after she moved into my apartment on Corso Vittorio near the river. I'd had two wives but no children. Now that I'd found a woman I thought I could stay with, I would have liked to have children, but Hannah was adamant. "How could I bring up a child? Tell him about the camps? Make him drunk on the milk of Auschwitz? I see what happens to my sister's children. How fearful they are without knowing why. My cats are enough. My cats and you...." She lurched up in the tub and grabbed at my arm.

"You're getting soap all over me," I laughed, but she didn't let go, looking at me with green glinting mermaid eyes. "I shouldn't let you care for me this way. It's too good. Too much what I want. What if you leave me?"

"I won't," I murmur. "Why do you tell yourself sad stories? The nightmare is over. Let yourself trust."

"I've lost everything—my language, my family. I can't lose you."

"Stop it. Stop yourself. It's over now." I found myself shaking her. My hands holding her shoulders covered with soap.

"Our neighbor offered me a place to hide," she went on, holding the thread of her memory. "In her cellar. But my mother wouldn't think of letting me go. She stood rubbing her hands on her apron and looking up at the sky, waiting for a sign while God spit on her."

"You're so angry." I pulled her even closer, ignoring the

water soaking my clothes. "But still you sleep with a piece of your mother's embroidered apron beneath your pillow." She nodded. It was all she had left. I didn't tell her then, but I had a plan to frame that scrap of mother love and surprise her by hanging it above her desk.

The irony is that I couldn't stand the burden. I stood it for many years and I can't say they were unhappy years, but it was too much—to be there, to be always available to her. Always soothing, helping. Twenty years of married care. It was too much. I felt mean, small, but I couldn't respond anymore to the endless physical ailments. I didn't only have to sympathize, I had to talk her down. So brave as a child but now always fearful, lost in the streets in front of our house, expecting cancer, heart attacks. She had fears about losing our apartment, fears about travel. Once she had to get off the train when we were going for a preview of one of my films.

I'm not sure when it started with Claudia. At first it was sort of a joke. When I was making my film, *Journey into Madness*, about a schizophrenic girl, the actress I had cast as the therapist had no breasts, but my dentist's wife Claudia's were superb. I asked Claudia to double in a few key shots and she was just vain enough to let me display her body. Or maybe she was impressed that I was a famous director.

One of my films had just won an Academy Award for best foreign film of the year. I now had the unexpected luxury of being able to make whatever films I wanted. I wrote a script about a girl who is in crisis after a terrible automobile accident. When she is brought to the hospital, she is in a near-catatonic state, unable to move or speak; wrapped in mummy bandages, no longer struggling. Only if you looked closely you could see the skin of her mouth quiver. A Picasso world where eyes, noses, teeth hung crazily, known but unrecognized. And all seen in a glaring light making everything shiny and smooth. Metallic voices. Words without meaning spoken by puppets. No warmth anywhere.

Her parents visit and seem just as frozen. Rich, spoiled people who couldn't be bothered. Blind to her suffering. Making social chitchat with her doctors. Too bad she couldn't be like her younger sister, they simper, a perfect, beautiful, gifted child.

I had a perfect sibling too. Although of course I loved my brother, he always outclassed me; he was always more handsome, humble, modest, and appealing. Despite my successes in writing and directing, my brother was always my mother's favorite.

So I put my heart into this film. I was daring. I wanted to convert the girl's inner world to something an audience could experience. I wanted to make them see the sudden shifts. Frame 1: A child plays in the schoolyard. She is looking at the fence. Seeing it with the exactness of a camera. Frame 2: But now she doesn't recognize it. The singing children become prisoners. She cries in anguish. The school grows immense, and presses against her. The children are like ants. She shakes the grating, trying to get out.

I needed to show how the strangeness descends on the girl. Children are skipping rope. Suddenly one grows large as a lion, her features distorted. One, two, buckle my shoe. The girl is like Alice in a more dangerous Wonderland. Sometimes she fights the distortions, but more often she thinks of succumbing to what she calls the System, feels as if she is whirling on an infinite plane, crushed by the pitiless light. She wanders lost in an astral cold, terrified. She feels that if she sinks far enough into the System, she will stop feeling terror. I use painters to help me imagine her world: Dali with his bleak planes and distorted objects.

While I was shooting the film, I thought of my mother unable to bear any more of her voices as she was dragged deeper and deeper into her madness.

I thought of Hannah, too, making my own connections between the Gestapo guards and the elaborate punitive rules imposed on the schizophrenic girl by the System. Hannah described the inventive cruelty of the concentration camp matrons and the rage they inspired. The girl in my film has similar rages which I imagined in red tumor-like shapes, cancerous flowers, huge red mouths pulsing with the desire to eat, white stamens stark against the red like a Bosch painting. Some shapes with legs and arms kicking or striking. Some in the act of swallowing.

"I hate everyone," the girl says. "I want to blow up the world. Steal people's brains and leave them as robots obedient to my will." Her psychiatrist sits beside her, arm lightly around her shoulders and for the first time the frozen nature of things begins to thaw; she feels warmth. The therapist's breasts became crucial to the character's development and the relationship between the girl and her therapist in the film: big soft breasts that you could sink into like a pillow. Lying with her head on her therapist's breasts and pretending to nurse, the girl gradually recovers.

The therapist with Claudia's body tells her not to be afraid: she will be protected by her new mama. But the System doesn't let her go so easily. Objects begin to take on a life of their own. The jug with a blue flower asserts itself, comes towards her aggressively. Turning away, she sees a table, a chair—both alive (Alice's *Wonderland* again).

The actress playing the therapist was brilliant. While she held the girl, she would whisper that "she" had a lovely clean body. The therapist always referred to the girl in the third person because hearing the word "you" would send the girl into a panic. Making this come alive on film, I was both the good warm breast and the baby wanting relief. Embarrassing for a grown man to admit, but secretly, making that film before I left Hannah, I was trying to lessen my burden by making it a refuge.

When the girl feels the bond between herself and her therapist, the whole world starts to glow, warmth flooding her body. She feels the therapist's loving concern. She allows the therapist to feed her and will only take food from her hands.

I made a glowing light suffuse the scene, tinged it with rose—not corny the way it is when the cowboy rides off into the sunset but real and warm space—details of beauty: birds, sand, water. I wanted my audience to see it the way the girl did, suddenly waking to a different world, warm, filled with love. My plan was ambitious. I meant it to rival the great films and to an extent I think I succeeded. But though the reviews were good, people weren't excited by it; it was too subtle—or maybe I was aiming too high.

There are different ways of telling the story of Hannah and me that make me more or less culpable. What, for instance, if my wish for children had become overpowering and Claudia had said she would have one? She sometimes said she wanted one—a little me. But was Claudia really serious? I don't know. It would be just for the purpose of the story. What? Didn't you know that writers always mix fiction and fact?

I don't want to seem like a cad. Even after I "left" Hannah to be with Claudia, I visited Hannah every day for lunch or supper. And at the same time I tried to show her how foolish she was to hang on to me. Why didn't Hannah enumerate my flaws, my defects of character, my narcissism, my egotism, and say to hell with you? Hadn't her life experiences convinced her that there is no everlasting love?

"No, Renzo," she would say, shaking her head. "It is my reason to keep on living."

That's the sort of statement that scared me silly. After surviving Auschwitz was she going to die for love? More cruelly, was I killing her? She seemed to fall into fragments like a broken mirror. But listen, her state wasn't just because of me. Wasn't I the one who encouraged her to work, to put herself back together through her own efforts? In our early years together I read everything she wrote—all those stories about her childhood in the village. I encouraged her to tell the truth about her mother. She was a sainted martyr, yes, all right, turned to soap the first day, but she was also narrow-minded and punitive—always trying to press Hannah into an iron mold, ready to cut off her feet if they wouldn't fit. Just before they were expelled from their village her mother was trying to find a husband for her—at twelve years old.

For years I supported Hannah while she wrote all day, and I read every page in the evening. She never could wait until the next day. And then I took her stories into my heart and gave them new life in films. The village life lent itself to cinema. Colorful and full of a variety of characters. I combined the strongest stories. Hannah helped me with the screen plays. It brought us closer. My favorite story was based on her father—a kosher butcher who had only a donkey to draw his cart. His wife continually berates him for being a bad provider. Then one day he finds an emaciated horse and, full of joy, brings it back to his family, where the poor animal succumbs despite the children's frantic efforts to save it. People loved these stories; they were quite successful both in print and on the screen. Without me Hannah might not have found the courage to start.

I swing forward and backward in time. So many hours and minutes of peace.

"What are you doing?" she asked me one Sunday morning in our mythic beginning when she saw me stirring eggs in the frying pan.

"Making one of my specialties," I said.

"If you're trying to scramble them, turn the heat up." She laughed, seeing me in my apron, thinking I didn't know how.

"Go away," I said. "There isn't room for two. I can barely turn around. I'll call you when it's ready."

"Are you really doing this?" she asked me. Back then, not many men could be seen in the kitchen. I shooed her out and went back to my stirring. I actually enjoyed the feeling of the egg against my spoon. If you stir over a very low heat, it slowly thickens and becomes ambrosial. Its slowness was like my patience in dealing with Hannah. I called her in and served the eggs. Then I took her on my lap. She slanted her eyes at me suspiciously but she let me offer her a spoonful.

"One for you," I said, "and one for me. Isn't it delicious?"

"You're spoiling me," she said though she kept on eating. When she finished I sang her a little lullaby. I hadn't planned either to cook, or to sing—they came naturally and I was encouraged because she let herself relax and enjoy them. She reminded me of a wild kitten that lurked in the tall grass near the back door of our family villa outside of Todi. Constanza, our cook, would put out milk for her, milk the little one would only drink after we retreated into the dark depth of the house.

"Trust me," I said to Hannah, rocking her gently. "You can trust me." I'm not sure even now if that was true. Then I carried her back to bed and stroked her all over for a long time before entering her. She let me take care of her and she blossomed.

After I left, I still helped her. I helped her get other jobs writing scripts and then a few long feature articles for a glossy mass-market magazine. I remember her pride when the first article came out under her byline. She wanted to write about deviants: homosexuals, transsexuals, beggars—or female creativity. Her boss wasn't interested. He kept shunting her onto more anodyne topics. He was the typical chauvinist male, puffing big cigars and blowing smoke in her face.

When I moved out to live with Claudia, near Hannah's and my apartment, he tried to lure Hannah into bed with the subtlety of a Roman bus. When I came over for lunch, Hannah would tell me the latest outrageous things he'd done. She was a great mimic. "This is how he looked," she said one particularly upsetting day, puffing out her chest to look at her watch. 'I have two hours away from the office. Let's not waste it, let's fuck.'"

"Did he really say that?"

"And pushed against me with his erection. He's a pig."

"If he bothers you again, I'll speak to him. I'm still your husband."

"He knows you don't live with me anymore," she said accusingly, then immediately cancelled the accusation with a smile. "To soothe myself I made love with Carlos."

"Isn't he gay?" I'd asked, surprised.

"He wanted to help, he was very tender, we stayed in bed for hours."

I didn't like hearing these things but I put on a tender expression and held her hand. My friends thought I was crazy. I should make a clean break. They couldn't understand our lunch dates—every day for twenty years! In the end it was Claudia I broke up with.

These days, when people ask "How are you?"—in their cheerful ignorant way—I want to give them the suit I read about, the one that scientists put on young doctors to help them understand what the aging body feels like. How it drags you down. It was ingenious: there were even glasses that fogged your eyes and weights that made moving exhausting and gave you pains in your joints.

People say age encroaches gradually, on little fog feet, as it were, tiptoeing along the veins and arteries until suddenly one morning you wake up and see death grinning at you over the counterpane. But the worst aspect of aging, the one you don't speak about if you are unlucky enough to suffer it, is what happens to your mind.

In the beginning Hannah and I joked about my forgetting phone numbers, book plots, restaurant names. Even though she was so much younger, she claimed to be forgetful too. She wasn't though, and more and more her whole existence was taken up by Remembrance.

Lists she told me, make lists. But wait. Did I tell you that I was married for twenty years to Hannah before I left to live with Claudia, and then that I spent another twenty years visiting Hannah every day for lunch? I kept it up until she had a nearly fatal heart attack and I asked her to let me come back. It's amazing, don't you think? That she would forgive me and let me come back? But there was also humiliation. I was so diminished. And despite her heart attack, from which she quickly recovered, she was so much stronger.

The other day I bought her a beautiful book that I noticed in the window of a bookstore next to our palazzo, an early edition of Petrarch's sonnets. I put papers in to mark the sweetest love songs—the ones I could no longer sing. She took it back, and I'm sure she apologized to the bookstore owner; told him about her poor husband who can't find his way in the world anymore; who didn't grasp the impossible price. How humiliating. I fear it is just the beginning.

Yesterday I tried to give her five euros to help with the rent and she patted my cheek. "Thank you, Renzo," she said, "how sweet," the way you'd thank a child who gave you play money.

I went into my studio and cried. Opened one of my books and saw the list of my titles, my poetry, my films, and my honors. I re-read and fondled the framed awards and statuettes: the Oscar from Hollywood, the Golden Palm from

Cannes, the two Golden Lions from Venice, and the one I was most proud of, the *Sol Plaatje* award for my poetry. That cheered me but I still felt confused about the details of our life. Who paid the bills? The rent? Was Hannah in control? Of course not. I started to laugh. All I had to do was stay calm and the facts came back to me. I was the one who paid the bills and planned our finances. I had ever since our early days. My God, I taught her everything she knew. I sat her down every month and we went over the checkbook together. She hated doing it and the balance was always slightly off. But finally she had it down well enough.

I repeat like a litany the ways I encouraged Hannah's strengths. How I kept on urging her to write more about her village and her childhood; read her drafts, corrected her Italian, and finally, how I taught her to fall in love with natural beauty, the woods and streams. Despite the poverty it seemed like the Garden of Eden before the expulsion of Adam and Eve by the flaming angel with his sword.

I loved her village stories and I urged her to go further and write a memoir—everything else had been in the third person—about the expulsion and transport. I wanted to do a film about it and suggested she interview her neighbors, see how much they understood of what had happened. She wasn't sure she could.

"Not one of the women raised a finger to help us," she said. "They just stood by on the edge of the road and stared as the Nazis—some of them their husbands and sons—drove us like cattle going to market, beating us with sticks. Some of the women even joined in, throwing stones, people who'd sat in my mother's kitchen just days before or gossiped with her on market day."

I could see the scene begging me to shoot it. A flashback to the market with the piles of luscious fruit, grapes, pears, and melons, and the two girls holding hands as they looked or picking up the pennies that the horse traders sometimes threw to get them out of the way. Then I cut to her friend, staring along with the other women, tears in her eyes.

One day in the early sixties, urged on by me and buoyed by the success of her first novel, *Nobody Could Love You,* she got up the courage to visit her village. We boarded the Orient Express from Vienna to Romania. Hearing German on the train made her shiver.

"Tickets please," the conductor said, bending towards us.

She turned away, pressing herself against me, clinging, my arm around her. I tried to imagine how German sounded to her after that ride in a cattle car as a child of twelve. How all trips now are tainted—she still gets sick anytime she has to travel—and all sounds in that guttural language are curses. Even the raucous schoolboys in the next car are a threat. I wondered whether I had made a mistake.

When we arrived in the village with our handheld video camera, the villagers clustered around us. Hannah had brought a small icebox for a friend of her mother's, the only one she remembered. Her village had just gotten electricity, powered by boys taking turns on a bicycle. The villagers were excited by the gift but not particularly grateful—and she was right: they showed a complete lack of curiosity about what had happened to her family.

Hannah remembered several of the women, quite old now, by their gestures or a feature—a mole, a way of speaking. She had brought things for their children. "How is your mother?" one elderly woman asked her, as though she had not seen the soldiers driving them out, her mother wailing. Willed blindness, Hannah called it.

"When we were driven through the countryside with bare feet in the winter," she told me after the old woman had moved on, "our feet covered with chilblains, bleeding, putrid, most people turned away. Only a few threw pieces of bread from their windows, and then quickly shut them."

I wanted to show the blindness of the villagers alongside their welcoming hugs—the split between kindness and indifference to a brutal reality. I still fancied myself a therapist, showing Hannah how to trust. I was blind to the hurt I caused. I'd always felt the need to take care of the women in my family, my mother, my little sister.

Uneasy at first, Hannah soon wanted to look for her hut among the picturesque houses clustered around a central well. The houses were rough and unadorned, made of wood, with thatched roofs. Hers was nowhere to be found, though we searched the alleys where chickens and pigs rooted and scratched.

"These are palaces compared with mine," she said, as I trailed her with my camera. "Ours had so many holes in the roof we might as well have been out in the rain." She took a deep breath here, almost as if she were calling up a life force, and then went on. "You can imagine the eight of us jammed together in one bed. Papa and Mama in their bed behind a sheet where we could hear the noises of lovemaking. We listened with acute interest, just the way we watched the farm animals rutting. Dogs with their tongues hanging out spilling moisture, their red penises searching for the bitches' hole. After seeing two horses mate—the stallion so huge and impressive, I masturbated for the first time. From then on I was intensely interested in my brothers' morning erections." She laughed and pressed my hand.

I loved picturing her as a Rousseauian savage, barefoot, her clothes triple-patched, watching sex without neurosis. I exaggerated her freedom. There were always the straightened clothes, the harsh scrubbing of neck and face, the sharp tongue, the ill-tempered pronouncements of what a girl could and should do. Hannah was willing to have me bring out the earthy rebelliousness of her life in the village, but she always circled back not just to the Nazis but to her mother: sometimes blaming her for waiting so passively to be saved; at other times recalling with dreadful precision every slap and harsh word her mother had ever spoken.

When we first slept together, she told me afterwards, she was thinking of what her mother would have said. "She would have hated everything I've done since she died," she said with a crooked smile that rose slightly on only one side, giving her a lopsided look, half indulgent, half angry.

"Aren't you exaggerating?" I asked her.

"Look," she counted on her fingers. "The worst was that I married a *goy*. Second, that I've given up my religion, or at least she'd think I have. I don't go to temple not even to say *kaddish*. Then I don't have children. At least there would have been some hope because they'd be Jewish. And," she reached her pinky, "she would certainly hate my cats. All eight of them. Animals were for food, not to have as pets. She'd be scandalized that I let them lie in bed with me, and drink a little milk from my saucer while I'm having my latte. Even the way I spend my time writing. It was enough for her that I learned Hebrew, taught by an ugly old man who switched my legs when I was slow to answer."

When Hannah first met her, my mother was at the piano playing Chopin. "What beautiful music," Hannah said shyly, "and such an elegant woman. I can't imagine growing up in a place like this. Paintings of ancestors, tapestries, oriental rugs."

Our family villa was at the edge of the Borghese Gardens, surrounded by ancient pines. I remember how excited I was to have these two beloved women in one room. My mother was so gracious, going to Hannah and kissing her on both cheeks.

All my life I've been a romantic—at least since the age of three, when I told my mama I was going to marry her when I grew up. The energy for each love glowed inside me like a warm beating heart. But in proportion to the beauty I saw in each beloved woman, my disillusionment when it came was total: sometimes it was something seemingly trivial like a lover's laugh that suddenly became ribald, turning my beloved from a princess into a whore.

But there was never anything like that with Hannah. What I fell in love with was partly the image of myself in her mysterious green eyes: savior, caretaker, magician. How could I keep that up without destroying my substance, without being eaten from the inside? A therapist might have said I was caring for her like a mother, but I don't think that would have helped me keep it up. The weight of it was crushing. Claudia was the way out. Claudia, my dentist's wife, often helped out as his assistant, though it seemed to me she was as bored and hostile to him as I was. My teeth, though white and even, were soft and riddled with cavities. I could imagine some therapist peering into them looking for my secrets. I often fixed my eyes on her full breasts when she bent close to me to hand her husband some instrument. I convinced myself she was unhappy and fantasized about taking her breasts in my mouth, distracting myself from whatever torture her husband was engaged in.

When I first wrenched myself away from Hannah, I started a journal with the purpose of keeping track of how she was adjusting: taking vital signs. I sniff the pages and the book comes alive—slightly acrid, dusty. It falls open on a shock that I received one night back then: I had been lying in bed in our apartment—Hannah was staying with a friend next door while we figured out our living arrangements. Claudia was away somewhere with her mother. When I heard someone fumbling with a key outside my front door, I felt like a fool for not buying a triple lock. All Romans knew you had to have at least a dead-bolt. My lock was ridiculously easy. Child's play. I sat up just as the door swung open. In that instant I had a vision of guns firing, blunt instruments, death.

"It's me," Hannah said softly. My heart was beating madly. As I held my hands against it to quiet it, I remembered I hadn't taken back her key. I'd given it to her for emergencies. In a flash she was beside me, arms around me, pulling me down to the bed. "Hold me," she said between sobs, "please hold me." I stroked her hair.

"You can't do this, Hannah," I told her. "You know you shouldn't be here. Or were you torturing yourself with the thought of seeing us together, me and Claudia?"

"This is my home," she hiccuped. "See, I feel better already." I undid her arms.

"Please," she said hugging me to her. "Let me lie down with you."

"No, I can't, *can't* reward you for..." I wanted to say for bad behavior but I knew she'd be crushed.

"Oh, don't be so sanctimonious," she said giving me a punch on the shoulder. "What can she give you that I can't? You know I'd do anything just to be with you."

"Hannah, we've gone over this so many times. Sooner or later you'll see it's the only honest way and you've always prized hon..."

"Oh, for heaven's sake, stop," she moaned, kissing my face. I had the weird thought that she wanted to bite me in the throat. That she was swinging from love to hate.

"But why Claudia?" she asked. "She's the sort of woman we used to make fun of. Not an idea in her head, just big boobs to redeem her. When you chose her for those body shots in your film we laughed about it together, and then...."

I was getting impatient and wanted to get back to sleep. But I knew she was suffering and I thought she had a right. Besides, though she seemed rational, I knew that when she was alone again, she'd fall apart and start castigating herself, certain that she had no chance of winning me back, that I was angry.

"I need you both," I said wearily. "I don't want to loose either of you. You know that. Now go back and get some sleep.

If your friend wakes up and finds you gone, she'll worry." She dropped her hands and pulled away peering at me in the moonlight like an angry ghost. "I'm not mad at you. It's just a lapse. Everyone has them once in a while ... *ogni tanto puo suc-cedere*." I stressed the "once in awhile."

After she left I thought about how it often happens that when we are most frantic about losing love, we do just the thing calculated to irritate or even drive away the loved one. Write the letter, send an envoy, call up on one pretext or another. Hannah was no different.

When she first found out about me and Claudia—which was just after we'd bought a vacation home on the beach at Forte de Marmi—she was driven mad by the idea that I took Claudia there and that I had stopped making love to her, Hannah, because Claudia provided better sex. She would sit on the sofa in provocative poses or I'd find her in bed in a tight corset or lacy underwear with a slit at the crotch.

"Why do you wear this silly thing?" I asked her annoyed that she was ruining the spontaneity I prized. And she started to cry. When I mentioned this to Claudia she rebuked me for humiliating Hannah. And of course Hannah was right, in a way. Claudia *did* give me another kind of sex. Sex that had no strings attached, that wasn't a declaration of eternal love or even of love that was going to last until next week. It was just a good fuck with an easy-going woman, whereas sex with Hannah involved recriminations, tears, and always a nagging sense of guilt that would make me review all the things I had done for her and how I would always love her.

"Why are you leaving me?" she asked over and over.

"I'm not leaving. I want to live in two houses that's all. I don't want to be a hypocrite. I want you both. That's just how I am."

This was the era of my power over Hannah. All her being was concentrated on bringing me home. Before, she had always been loving; now she had a sort of desperation that made her eyes shine and her cheeks redden. I liked the way, when I called to tell her I wanted to see her, she dropped everything, even threw people out of the apartment. I hated myself for indulging myself this way but I was virtually addicted. I kept telling her to forget me though I knew she couldn't.

I am still fascinated by splits between kindness and hate, whether among Hannah's villagers, soft-spoken American Southerners, or myself. I used to try and talk to Claudia about this.

"Of course people are capable of both," Claudia snorted, "why do you worry about such things. Don't be naïve. Aren't there enough things to worry about? Wait until you are kidnapped like Aldo Moro."

Claudia was obsessed by his capture. Every night she was glued to the television while talking heads described the position the government should take. Should they negotiate with the *Brigate Rosse*, pay them what they asked, or should Moro himself urge them to stand firm and if necessary die a martyr? When he was assassinated she was horrified. I think she was convinced it was an elaborate game of chicken.

Now that I'm nearly ninety years old, I wake up in the late morning when the sun enters directly and I'm not sure where I am: in her old apartment or mine. For a moment after waking up, I'm not sure. But then I take ownership again of the terraces loaded with flowering plants, pots of geraniums, huge soft ferns, cacti, and the view over the city, the rooftops. I watch the gulls circling, crying out like children, or sometimes like cats in heat on a summer night. A gull has laid her eggs on the jutting roof just below us, protected by a raised drain.

"What are you doing?" Hannah asks from the terrace door, "I didn't know where you were."

"Did you think I had vanished, flown away?" Jumping off the terrace does have its attractions, doing away with myself before I lose the ability to remember.

A week later the eggs hatch and three fluffy balls of gray tumble over each other, trying to walk on the curved roof tiles. I can watch for hours, feeling the warmth of the late spring sun on my back. The parents take turns flying off, spreading powerful white wings and returning with food that they regurgitate for the little ones, who signal their hunger by pecking at their parents' bills.

I'm as fascinated as if I were watching some earth-shattering event: the pope at Easter on the Vatican balcony addressing the crowds. I stare as a small snake emerges from the parent's craw and is swallowed by the least vigorous of the chicks. He can't quite get it all down and one of his siblings grabs the end and swallows it until only the tip is showing. The game continues until finally the stronger one succeeds in getting it all in.

I fell some months ago and broke my hip. There were complications and I found myself condemned to my bed for two months of hell. Who could have ever imagined that reading would take so much effort? Our attic apartment was packed full of books. In the little room that opens onto the first terrace, they run from floor to ceiling—all the English classics, Dickens, Scott; the French, Balzac, Victor Hugo, Rimbaud, Becket, Sartre. My eyes stop at Sartre's *Nausea*—that would describe pretty well the sick state of my soul. In past days, which I can now hardly remember, I would dip into it just to show myself my basic healthiness.

Hannah says our early married life was too calm for me to tolerate—like a peaceful lake. There is some truth in that, particularly when I was young, but she doesn't seem to realize how much of myself I had to submerge and leash. She had experienced the worst human beings can do to each other.

How could I subject her to petty squabbles? I feel now as if I am coming undone, part by part. My eyes tire after a few minutes and if I leave a book for a few days, I don't remember who the characters are.

Hannah cares for me exquisitely these days but I some-times hear her on the phone with her friends, speaking in a funereal voice.

"Yes, it is so complicated now. My husband isn't well, poor thing. He broke his hip you know. I can't leave him alone."

Sometimes she can still be playful as a kitten. My old friend Ernesto came over for lunch with his new wife, Elena, and Hannah cooked her mother's pancakes—some-thing between a latke and a quiche. What impressed me was how she sang in the kitchen and how strong she looked, car-rying the heavy bowl of soup and then afterwards digging out the gelato in big chunks, ignoring their insistence that they couldn't eat another bite, not pulling away from me when I put my arm around her and patted her thigh.

After three glasses of white wine I don't feel eighty-eight. I see the young wife studying me. She knows our story from books that each of us has written, films we've made, gossip in the news, and she looks as if she is trying to figure out what attractions this old coot has, could have had. I stare into her eyes, mine still a penetrating green, or at least after the wine I think so...windows of the soul. I slap Hannah's thigh again. Elena asks about my film, *Journey into Madness*. I tell her I saw the girl's journal introduced by a French psychoanalyst and immediately felt drawn to it for a film. This analyst had saved the girl and sent her to school to study medicine. When the analyst died, the girl killed herself. She needed a lot of love.

"I was a laureate in medicine myself," I tell the young wife. "Then came film and poetry. I didn't want to give up making films, but when I turned eighty no one wanted to give me a job anymore. It was too risky. No insurance company would insure the film. What if I died halfway through? No, just like that I was finished." I pause, hearing the self-pity in my voice. "Well, life goes on. We can fight aging to the best of our powers ... as Dylan Thomas said: '*Do not go gentle into that good night; rage, rage against the dying of the light.*'"

I can't stop trying to interest the young wife. She has something sensual about her mouth that attracts me.

"Every morning," I tell her, "I go to my bookcase and take out a book, Tolstoy or Dostoyevsky or, better still, one of the metaphysical poets—John Donne writing sonnets in his coffin—and read a couple of pages. Let it settle in my mind as a keynote for my day. These are all books I have read before, of course."

"Oh," she says politely, as if I am a new animal in the zoo—one of those bears with matted fur and bald patches. I must say I still have a full head of iron-gray hair, and I cover my old bones with a good suit from Armani, the one luxury I permit myself besides my daily tub of gelato.

Elena is interested in the fact that I moved back in with Hannah after her heart attack. "It was time," Hannah laughed. "After so many years apart. Now it's a backward race to the finish line. Who will arrive first? I know it was hard for me to return to consciousness when I had my heart attack," Hannah says, "I was in such a deep, still place. I lost the ability to talk for a week. But now I am glad."

Glad probably isn't the right word. Part of the truth is that she is afraid to go too far from home now, always watching for the telltale symptoms.

I am becoming obsessed with aging; I feast on others' misfortunes—wanting I suppose to prepare myself for whatever comes next. I heard the news of another old friend's illness, Lucian. I hadn't seen him in years—since Hannah had quarreled with him over some gossip she had repeated about his family. Though Hannah and Lucian had once had a deep friendship, both of them were too stubborn to make the first move to reconcile. I had a fantasy of making peace between them while there was still time. He had multiple infirmities, more serious than mine.

Adolescence prepares our parents for our departure, disease—the more painful the better—readies us for death. Fine thought, but still I can't imagine the world without my consciousness. I am furious at the idea of it going on without me. Horrified and furious! I can't understand how some people can throw a farewell party, invite all their friends, and then retire to their room with a deadly cocktail or a gun.

I wondered how Lucian was taking his decline and decided to visit him. I called a taxi and asked the driver to come up and help me down. I chose a time when Hannah had gone out to the market on Campo dei Fiori and was going to meet a friend for coffee before coming home. Sitting where she could look at the piles of glowing fruits and leafy vegetables, cheering herself with plenty.

In the taxi, I recalled my last visit with Lucian—him telling Jewish jokes and laughing at them, playing up his Brooklyn roots while his wife Gabriella sat quietly, every inch an aristocrat, with the slight curl of an ironic smile. I had taken him for granted, I guess, thinking that he'd always be there so I didn't have to hurry. But I realized in the taxi that he was probably the only one still alive of the filmmakers who left Hollywood for Mexico to escape McCarthy.

He and my poet friend George were gone ten years, hiring themselves out as carpenters. When George came back to the States, he won a Pulitzer Prize. Lucian came to Rome—he couldn't film anymore except under a pseudonym—and married Gabriella. He liked to tell how her shrink had said he was the best of her suitors. He was very handsome in a Jewish sort of way, dark wavy hair, full lips. I should have taken a tape-recorder and recorded him—last of the old Reds. Reds on the black list. Where did all that fire and passion go?

I got such a shock when Lucian opened the door and stepped forward to embrace me. A wool watch cap on his head, his face grizzled. Well, he's an old man and his head gets cold, but then I saw the open bathrobe with a bag of urine dangling between his legs and a white slice of diaper. We talk. He insists on pushing his walker down the hall to the kitchen and bringing a glass of wine.

"Let me do that," I beg him, walking behind him. Wondering whether I could hold him if he falls. He condescends to let me bring in a bowl of olives and some napkins. Gabriella is depressed and he's not sure she'll join us. But she does and she is wearing a beautiful Chinese robe. Holding her elegant head high, arms outstretched to greet me. I've brought her a catalogue of the Pre-Raphaelite show.

Lucian's doorbell rings and to my surprise it's Ernesto and Elena. Gabriella looks at the pictures while Lucian monologues about his life to the young wife. I'm jealous—I thought she was just interested in Hannah and me. Is she going to be promiscuous then, collecting old codgers for some project of hers—Communists in the Forties? Reds on the blacklist? Lucian is wearing a hearing aid and can only hear me from the left side. Gabriella tries to comment occasionally on the paintings but he ignores her. She shrugs.

"He can't hear me anymore," she says with a note of desperation. No wonder she spends much of her time in bed.

Back home the gulls are circling, giving their sunset calls. I love the inexorable progress, the same year in, year out, from the blue-green elegant eggs kept warm by mother and father in turn, to the newly hatched chicks stumbling when they try to walk on their big black feet; later, the adolescents unfolding their wings for practice, not yet aware of their power. And then one day they take off on a favorable current.

But what I'm really jealous of is that they have no foreknowledge of death.

Do you ever wake up in the morning so irritated that you scream if your psychic wound is touched by anyone—particularly by someone dear to you who is trying to help—and look for an object on which to discharge your anger? Of course you do. Kick the dog, curse the government.

In my case I wake up angry with Hannah. She won't sleep in my bed anymore. She just puts me to bed like a child, holding me until I fall asleep, then moves into the other room. She says I snore. It occurs to me that she humiliated me when our friend was here with his new wife. Hannah asked me to collect the plates and I couldn't hear her. There must have been some conversation going on that interfered with my hearing aid, and I handed her the salt and pepper.

"No", she said in a cranky voice, "not those." Then more gently, "Why don't you turn up your ears?"

The young Elena had looked at me sympathetically and I blushed purple. That wasn't at all the way I wanted to attract her attention! The truth is I love it when Hannah cuddles close to me and strokes my thinning hair. I love it way more than I am willing to admit, but my penis is ashamed that it no longer has a voice in what goes on. It lies quiet and limp between us—sometimes rousing a little—Hannah is still a handsome woman even though her magnificent braid is gray not gold.

I've been trying to write down things that are important to me—a storehouse for my memories. I tell Hannah I am working on a memoir. I don't tell her how difficult I find even recording my fleeting thoughts. My mind seems to take itself off on crooked little jaunts, mocking seriousness and relevance or even progression. Today for instance I am thinking about Lucian flaunting his urine in a plastic bag. If my penis is under-used and sad, think of how his must feel reduced to a waterspout. It took a certain kind of courage for him to show it off. Look, god damn you. You'll get there too soon enough.

At some point Gabriella brought in a photo of him from his twenties, slender with a hawk nose, thick black hair.

She wanted to remind me of what he'd been. Instead I found myself getting bored as he reviewed his life. I know, I know, you had a common-law wife in Mexico to console you for your exile—I picture her with fleshy dark thighs and enormous breasts, cooking huge skillets of refried beans, feeding him up, coddling him. Still, you left her, didn't you, even though you'd had a child? And when you came back you had to change your name, and none of your films are remembered—not your coming-of-age novel either.

Ah, yes that's what makes great areas of my brain flash red. The pain centers all firing at once as if I'd touched a red-hot pan. Ouch!

I worry that no one will remember me.

It's different with my older brother, Mario. Mario will probably die as if he were going on an expedition to the North Pole—afraid but excited at the adventure. If there is a cliff that you have to climb to reach posterity, he did it. I console myself that, except for certain geniuses, the rest will gradually fade out, interesting only to people like the young wife—didn't she say she was getting some kind of a degree at NYU?—peering with her large bright eyes into the murky past.

Hannah took me to see a special exhibit of ephemera at the museum of the city of Rome, Palazzo Braschi. We went in a taxi and I noticed she kept fingering her cell phone. Though she hates technology—she still writes on an old Olivetti and refuses categorically to get a computer—the phone means she can go a little further afield and still feel comfortably in touch with the *Ospitale*. The show was brilliant, everything made out of papier-mâché, huge intricate creations all meant to be destroyed after the festivity. I spent much of my time looking at images of death, such as a crowned skeleton presiding over ruins.

It was hard for me to imagine spending so much effort creating something that would be blown up a few hours after it was finished. I've struggled all my life to make something that would last. Would it be easier to let go if I believed in God? We had a housekeeper once, a peasant woman from the countryside whose son was killed in a fight with a rival gang in Naples. Most people would be depressed and grieving for months, but Argelide—aptly named after a heroine in Ariosto's *Orlando Furioso*—prayed for about a week, bringing her Bible to work and having murmured conversations with Lord Jesus and then resumed her serene expression.

"Signor, I know he's with our Lord," she told me. "I know he repented and was forgiven."

I can get as far as imagining a supreme being, having passionate conversations with a loving Father, prostrating myself with a certain self-satisfaction on the floor of Santo Spirito. But Heaven is so insipid. There is no way I would want to be in such a place. Singing out of tune in the heavenly choir. Angels poking each other with their wings each time I hit a wrong note.

Who am I fooling with my joking? Not myself certainly. I am terrified. Each flutter of my heart, incipient nausea, sweating on a cool day—any of these can convince me I am about to die. Since it happens to all of us, as the skeletons on the festival floats remind us, why this need to know when? To outwit the bony hand with its scythe?

I did notice something that cheered me up. A papier-mâché replica of a huge arch that was put up by Carlo V, Holy Roman Emperor, to celebrate his conquest of Rome in 1527. It was built just at our corner on Governo Vecchio, right where the old men sit in the morning gossiping and reading their papers in the little café that has the best *cornetti*. How delightful it would have been to watch from our terrace as the king progressed along the cobbled street to visit the pope. That's what I love about Rome. Every few feet there is a historical gem. I look at my watch. I've gotten through two hours of the morning. In another hour Hannah will put away her manuscript and take me for a walk. I have the thought that if death came to get me, she would frighten him off.

Today I was watching three adolescent gulls on the terrace next to ours. They were practicing flying. The biggest one tried first. Running across the tiles precariously near the edge, he lifted his wings and immediately was transformed from an ungainly creature in the wrong element to a thing of beauty. Flap, flap and he rises a foot above the roof, then subsides and folds his wings. His siblings try next. The wind comes up, blowing sharply from the East. I turn to put down our terrace umbrella. It tends to fall over in a strong wind even without a storm. Once, at the beginning of summer, it blew over and smashed into our bonsai tree. The pot cracked right down the middle and the tree toppled over, exposing its tangled roots. It could have hurt anyone sitting there.

That's how things work. You can't anticipate them. I turn the crank and the umbrella folds down. The smallest gull, the one I've noticed is always last when its parent comes with food, always standing at a respectful distance, is starting out quite near the edge, stumbling along and then—if he'd been a boy I'd say he feels a need to prove himself—flaps boldly and without warning tumbles over the edge. Wasn't ready, poor creature. I go in and tell Hannah that a gull has fallen.

"Don't go down, you'll just upset yourself," she says.

"Don't patronize me," I say and head for the front door. Making sure not to fall, I go cautiously down the steps to the creaky old lift. I hate using it by myself because it sometimes gets stuck between floors, and once we had to wait for over an hour for the mechanic. But at least Hannah knows where I am. If it takes too long she'll worry and check. Inside the lift I reprimand myself for my anxiety. I used to be confident. Now every potential disaster frightens me, from the collapse of the economy and the victory of that clown Berlusconi to the blister on my little toe that might turn into a life-threatening infection.

I walk—shamble would be more accurate—out the big front door that is getting almost too heavy to open—and see the gull, seemingly not injured at all, standing on the sidewalk in front of our palazzo. Like all young gulls he is a sort of fawn white. He cocks his head and looks at me with his red eye, then looks upward, as if wondering how he can get back. Our friend Arianne who lives on Campo di Fiori says that the fish man she uses on the square has a gull that comes every noon when the market is breaking up to collect his scraps.

I wish I'd brought something to offer him but I'm quite sure he wouldn't let me pick him up. He starts rushing at the wall flapping his wings, but only lifts a few feet. Then he waddles disconsolately down the street towards the café. Maybe he'll pick up some stale *cornetti*. Every few steps he tries another assault on the wall—a little the way an adolescent boy, powered by testosterone, might try to go against gravity. There was nothing more to do.

"Well?" Hannah asked when I came into the living room. I felt flooded by a sense of shame, as if I were the one running at the wall and failing to rise. Life is made up of so many tests.

"His wings look powerful," I said. "But he has always been a little smaller than his siblings. I guess he just wasn't ready. Maybe he was just trying to impress his mother." Hannah didn't laugh. She patted my hand, then sighed, and glanced down at her Olivetti. It was clear she wanted to get back to her work.

There was no point in going to my room and riffling through my aborted poems. I went back to the terrace and leaned over the wall. Our remaining gulls were napping between the red roof tiles, the mother sitting serenely on a chimney surveying the sky for threats to her offspring. After brushing off the tiny red spiders that ran along the edge and had adhered to my sweater, I leaned over a little further.

How easy it would be to simply tumble. Just by leaning over until your head pulled you down. Ever since I heard about the suicide of my friend Gina's daughter, I had wondered how she got the courage to jump out of her bedroom window. It was uncanny the way she'd made it a form of theater, dressing herself all in black with high heels, making herself up. I couldn't believe it at first when her mother, Gina, called us.

"I have some bad news," Gina said. "Bianca has jumped again. This time she made sure an awning wouldn't save her. She jumped from her bedroom window."

I signaled Hannah to pick up the extension. "The police woke me at five this morning and told me there was a girl down in the piazza. I ran into Bianca's room and saw at a glance the bed hadn't been slept in and the window was open, its white curtain billowing like a sail in the breeze…our bird had flown."

We had just seen Bianca a week before, taken her out to dinner in fact. Though she was still on crutches and in pain, she seemed so full of life, telling us that after jumping once, being seriously hurt and in a coma for weeks, and seeing all the people in the hospital who had lost limbs or had frightful wounds, she began to feel grateful for another chance at life. She wanted to move out of her mother's apartment on Campo dei Fiori and get a little place of her own.

"But don't you still need help?" I asked. Bianca still had a rigid corset under her clothes that made it almost impossible to reach or bend.

"My mother doesn't help me. She wouldn't even tie my shoes when I asked her the other day. She drinks you know. Seriously. And she resents the burden—told me this wasn't the way she'd planned her retirement."

We'd been friends with Gina for forty years or more, and apparently we didn't know her. She had always spoken of her daughter Bianca with cloying tenderness, insisting on calling her *micino*—kitten—although she was over thirty. Gina tried by every means to keep Bianca in the apartment. I had always thought it was Gina's fear of being alone after her pretty-boy husband left her. She still doted on him though he has re-married. Carlo had left her for a scholar of D'Annunzio—our proto-fascist poet—a handsome woman with jet black hair who reminds me of the sultry female in the Charles Addams cartoons. Gina has never been pretty but she has a keen mind laced with wit. Her satiric poems, posted on Pasquino's statue are legendary.

Well, here I am talking about Gina in a faintly superior tone of voice, perhaps even blaming her for wanting to keep her daughter near, for not wanting to be alone as she ages, when I myself would be devastated if I were *solo solito*. Isn't that why I asked Hannah to take me back? I like to think it was because of concern for her, wanting to be near her in case her heart went wild again. Her story of losing consciousness and then of losing the ability to speak scared me terribly. But my heart has its own jumpy rhythms and flutters. The big one could happen to me next time. My heart could clench up like a fist or go soft and floppy like a wilted cabbage. But is that a reason to anticipate by jumping?

Hannah would say absolutely not—under no conditions. It was a glorious sunny day, one that Tiepolo might have painted, when Primo Levi, a treasured friend of Hannah's, called her confessing that he felt depressed, and was thinking of suicide. I was surprised at how stern she was with him. Told him he had no right to think of it. Where would that leave her and the other Auschwitz survivors? She beat her head with her hands when she heard of his death.

I notice that I want to connect everything by ellipses, nothing separate, because it all runs together in my mind now, with things popping up, one leading to another. It doesn't seem to matter anymore exactly when or where... or at least that's what I tell myself. If I had to be exact, well, I couldn't go on.

This morning all I can think about are the clouds. I am sitting on the terrace in one of the canvas chairs. The bottom is torn, I notice, but don't get up to change my seat. So many things are getting to be too much trouble. Even brushing my teeth sometimes seems too much. Habits are breaking up. But the clouds are beautiful. Huge snow-white cumuli. One looks like a character in a children's cartoon with fat puffy arms and bottom. If I had grandchildren, I think I could get pleasure from watching them live, carrying on where I leave off. Now the gulls are circling in front of the clouds, white on white. Off to the left over the Palace of Justice, there is a shape that reminds me of the Jungfrau where we used to go for vacations when I was a boy, and where later, climbing with rope and pitons, I got away from the nastiness after Mussolini signed his pact with the devil. Black and white—the pure sky and the *Fascisti* down below.

Hannah brings me tea. She has a large green shopping bag with her.

"You're going out," I say accusingly.

"Just to the market. Don't worry." She turns my arm so that my watch is visible. "Not more than an hour. Back by noon and then we'll go out." She kisses the top of my head, caresses my hair. I have the impulse to tell her that I might not be here, wanting to frighten her, make her attend to me, watch me, cosset me. I can hear the lift going down, creaking like a freight train.

Late in the war, when I was in the Resistance with my remaining Jewish friends, we were always afraid of not coming back from a mission. I was lucky. Once, I was in the underground with Gabriella after her brother, Primo Levi, had been deported. She was carrying a huge green bag filled with antifascist leaflets. She used to walk all over Rome distributing them. They used her a lot because she didn't look Jewish. Unexpectedly the *Fascisti* closed the station and started to question people on the platform. One of them wanted to look at what she had, but she said it was a present for her grand-mother, and she was so much a lady, so dignified and proud…miraculously, he moved off. Back then, every moment of being alive was a victory.

Sounds of music from down on the street. Looking over the terrace wall I see a procession right beneath me with flags, people singing as they move along Corso Vittorio Emmanuele. There is a float with a woman and two lambs. Lambs—it must be the feast day of Sant'Agnese. On her birthday lambs are shorn and their wool made into the *pallia* the pope gives his archbishops. When I was small before my mother's death, the disaster that ended my childhood, I loved Sant'Agnese, the magnificent baroque church in Piazza Navona. I loved the intricate dance of its curves and the plunging horse plashing in Bernini's fountain in front.

My parents only went to church on special occasions like a baptism or a wedding, but at around the age of seven I became captivated by a book of saints' lives that I found in my father's library. I seem to remember it had a brief forward by Mussolini. By a strange coincidence, Mussolini had been my father's patient as an adolescent. *Il Duce* probably gave him the book as a gift. In a way, Mussolini was responsible for my going into film. My father took us to Switzerland after the Allies landed because he didn't want to be involved in Mussolini's Nazi Republic, and, to amuse ourselves, my brother and I attended a series of lectures by the great director Vittorio de Sico. That was the unofficial end of our medical studies though we stayed in the program for another two years to please our father.

How much of my life was dictated by a wish to please him! To make him proud I think I even entertained the idea of martyrdom for some heroic cause, like the saints in the little book.

Reading the leather bound Saints' lives, I learned that Saint Agnese was killed because she wouldn't marry the king's son—or was it because she refused to pray to pagan gods? She was beheaded because when she was tied to a stake, the fire wouldn't burn. Though I had no clear idea then of what it meant to be a virgin, I found myself oddly excited at the thought of Agnese being dragged naked though the streets of Rome to dirty her in some mysterious way. But it was Saint Lucie, the one with her eyes on a plate, that particularly fascinated me. How did her Roman torturers get them out, I wondered. If they gouged them with a metal instrument, wouldn't they have splattered? She looked so serene in the picture, and had another pair of eyes still in her head.

At the height of my religious fervor, I begged my parents to let me try out for the boys' chorus, the *voci bianche*. I had quite a good voice…very pure and strong. It wasn't until I was grown and reading about the priests molesting boys that I remembered being fondled by a young priest after Mass. It had bewildered me at the time because I actually liked the priest and looked up to him for his piety. Afterwards *I* felt guilty. As if I had somehow encouraged him to touch me that way. I was afraid something was very wrong with me. I hesitate even now to write it down. Not even Hannah knows about it.

What image of myself do I want to leave? Does it matter? Does anyone really care? If I look myself up on Google, there are three pages of references. At least fifteen of my film posters are displayed. All those sexy films—you can still order them and see them. Sophia Loren, Monica Vitti, Gina Lollobrigida, Anita Ekbert—I even had an affair with her. A woman that had all of Italy panting. I'd like to suggest that it was the serious aspect of my films that made me so successful, but it is really the more salacious ones for which I'm best known.

I remember the film where Vittorio Gassman comes to terms with being blind. How I wish I'd directed that one. You can't get much more serious than that.

I close my eyes and pretend I'm blind. I touch the edge of my desk, feel the smooth wood, white ash, to lighten my moods. The blotter is soft, no hint of its color. I infuse it with a deep blue. Then my hand moves to the cup where I keep my collection of pens and pencils, saved from years of travel. The Hotel Waldhaus pen has a particularly chunky body and there is the cushioned pen I got for my arthritis, but the others are indistinguishable.

I move my hand to my Luxo lamp. Perched like a small inquiring animal, its light is unavailable to me now. I think the first thing I would get if I lost my sight is voice recognition software. They say it isn't difficult, though the computer must be trained to recognize where words stop and start. You must be very patient and patience is not something I'm good at.

After a half hour of not being able to see, I stop. For a few minutes I actually feel blessed to still have my sight. I look out my window, gulping in the visual splendor of Borromini's bell tower in the distance. I should do that every morning instead of drinking coffee, which gives me stomach pains and makes my heart race.

For a moment I forget what day it is. It feels like Monday. The day housewives used to wash their clothes. But when I look at the calendar, I see that the days are marked off until Thursday, so it isn't Monday at all. It's Friday. It just occurred to me that when I talked about pretending to be blind, I should have put it in the past tense because how could I have written it down with my eyes shut? I am finding dates and tenses and calendars difficult. I even worried that I had gotten the dates wrong in my page about finding the book of saints' lives. When did Mussolini come to power exactly? I don't know anymore and I used to be so good at dates.

"Renzo," Hannah taps me on the shoulder and I look up hoping she has come to kiss me, to encourage me to face my day. "Do you remember that the *studentessa* with the big eyes is coming to interview you today?"

"I don't have any students anymore."

"I know, I know, I was just joking but she certainly acts

like one. You know who I mean—Ernesto's young wife, Elena. She has a project to do a video interview."

"Oh yes," I say but really I don't remember saying the young wife could come.

"On aging," Hannah adds kindly. "You should change your shirt. Wear the blue pinstripe. It brings out the color of your eyes." She goes to the closet and brings me the shirt and a fresh pair of khakis. Then leaves me to change. As though on cue, the doorbell rings just as I am zipping my pants.

"I'll get it," Hannah calls. You go into the *salòtto.*"

I wish she wouldn't tell me everything. I can still decide the best spot to be interviewed. I'm not that far gone. Not a child either. But she gets pleasure out of always being the one who knows.

It turns out that the interview is to be about what is beautiful in aging. How did I ever agree to this? Probably just because I like looking at a pretty woman, especially when she is looking back at me.

Elena is wearing a pink shirt that clings to her breasts. They are not big but sweetly shaped. I sigh and take up the paper she gives me. Instead of questions, there is just a repeated phrase: aging is beautiful because…

"Age isn't beautiful, it's horrendous," I say.

"Please," she pleads, looking at me with her big eyes. Her legs are as lovely as her breasts. Tanned, shapely.

"Age is beautiful," I go on, pleased with the idea of twisting the phrase to mean its opposite, "because you look at a girl and she doesn't see you.

"Age is beautiful because you don't remember the words of a song.

"Age is beautiful because you can't tie your shoes.

"Age is beautiful because you fall and break a leg. Here I look at her and smile. My smile is still good, I think. It underlines the wry humor in my responses.

"Age is beautiful because you talk and are not understood.

"Age is beautiful because you fix a telephone and it doesn't ring." Just as I say that the phone does ring and the young wife laughs. I wish I could think of a project that would have her visiting more often. It is Lucian calling me. I tell him to call back and look back at the paper.

"Age is beautiful because you piss your pants." No. That was too much. Over the line. She grimaces, no longer amused.

"*Basta*," I say. "Enough. Let's have some tea." Hannah, acting the part of secretary, had brought in the teapot. Reaching for it, I drop my cane. The young wife lunges towards it obviously afraid I'll crash, but I beat her to it.

"Don't worry, my dear. I've got it," I say, retrieving it awkwardly.

My head feels heavy, as though it is determined to pull me down, while my thighs are signaling distress at having to hold me back. Poor me. Trying to ignore my pains, I suggest to the young wife that she add some photos of me as a young man. I tell her where to look for the photo album on the high shelf near the door. I've shown enough bravado for one day. She mounts the little step-stool gracefully and pulls it down. The photos are black and white, slipped into black corners. I motion to her to sit beside me on the white couch and together we turn the pages.

"You were so handsome," she says.

"Were?" I tease, and she blushes. God, I was a lion... baring my teeth in a seductive smile. Thick dark hair. Sex seemed to radiate from my skin. She feels it too and my transformation bewilders her. I am like a desiccated insect, its color faded. Now it is all mental. Games for a failing man. Loose on the page is a recent photo that has slipped its moorings. I can see exactly how the bottom of my face has sunk and become gaunt, bones jutting out where there used to be plump glossy skin. I sigh.

"I've tired you," she says guiltily, putting her papers together.

After Hannah shows her out, I start thinking of couples I know where one is old and the other young, like Carlo Ponti and Sophia Loren. Power and Beauty living together and I no longer have either. She stayed with him her whole life and was with him when he died. Thinking about death depresses me and I go back to bed and sit there reading a magazine. Articles with pictures are easier for me when I feel this way. I pause at a picture of a beautiful little girl of around five, with cascades of ringlets. The caption is, "Was she killed by her mother?" How could anyone hurt this angelic being? Apparently, the mother's boyfriend didn't want her around. He felt she interfered with his plans and wishes. I always used to say that some people oughtn't to have children.

It's a cliché that having children is a blessing. Often when a couple is on the verge of separating, they'll have one "to bring them close again." But actually it is a huge strain, like driving an eighteen-wheeler over a bridge that hasn't been upgraded in years.

I never felt up to it. Playing with my nephews for a couple of hours was delightful but really all I could manage. I'm not boasting. It makes me sad that I felt so incapable.

After the war many of my friends went into analysis. It was a fad among intellectuals. Both Gabriella and Lucian were analyzed. They ended up getting married. Gabriella's shrink pronounced after meeting Lucian that he was the best of her suitors. I fantasized that it could help me find the perfect mate. Instead, my analyst seemed to be reading from a script, speaking with reverence of the Oedipus complex as the key that unlocked every neurosis including the one that stood in the way of my progress.

It's not that my relationship with my mother couldn't bear looking into—I was a manipulative, histrionic child and from early on I could wheedle almost anything out of her. It was the analyst's attitude that upset me. So knowing, so superior, as though he were a god, not a human being with ordinary flaws. Belief in Freud was at its peak. And if I ever objected to one of his interpretations, he would insist I was resisting.

"Don't you see zat?" He spoke Italian with a strong German accent, particularly clear on his consonants. "This it is part of ze transference onto me of feelings that you had towards your vather?"

I should have left. The truth is I had no transference to my analyst, not even a liking for him. If I'd liked him I might have accepted more of his interpretation. As it was, my image of myself suffered and I came away with a negative view of myself.

The analyst perceived right away that under my charm and warmth I was a somewhat selfish narcissist. I erase the word *narcissist* and leave the qualified *somewhat selfish*. *Narcissist* seems too harsh. His judgment of me still hurts. True, I didn't want a child to take a woman's attention away from me. But thousands of men probably feel the same way.

And by the time I found Hannah, wasn't she herself my mother-child in one? She, too, wanted total possession. She couldn't share me anymore than I could have shared her. She was damaged more grievously than most, a child who had suffered the unspeakable cruelty of the camps. But that only made it more challenging to save and nurture her. Every time I thought of something new to bring her, I felt as excited as I did when I was shooting a film or writing a poem and something snapped into place. And I loved the image of myself I saw in her eyes: liberator, magician of the possible.

When I met Hannah in her early twenties she had a rudimentary knowledge of Italian, spoke Romanian and Yiddish, and only knew enough Hebrew to pray. How it excited me in those early days and years to introduce her to art and the books I loved. At first she was hesitant. Her mother had rebuked her innumerable times for sitting in the house reading poetry instead of praying. She would tear the book from Hannah's hand. Angry at what she called her fantasies. Without poetry life would be insupportable, Hannah said, her head on my shoulder.

"Why didn't Mamma know that?"

She had forgotten all she knew in Auschwitz, even the songs. I felt I was participating in a rebirth.

I had no doubt about what I wanted to offer her first. I went right to Dante. I'd always felt that the fifth Canto of the *Inferno* was, though spiritualized, extremely erotic. I pictured reading it and then tumbling into bed. I drew her over to the couch and opened my book with its sensuous red leather cover. We sat shoulder to shoulder reading the wonderful stanza where the poet summons the lovers Paolo and Francesca to tell how they were undone by love. Their punishment of course is to never be separated, blown like morning doves by the wind. Francesca explains to Dante that when she and Paolo read about how the great lover Sir Lancelot kissed his beloved's longed-for smile, Paolo, Francesca's own love, lost restraint and "kissed me on the mouth, all trembling:"

> *Quando leggemo il disiato riso*
> *Esser baciato da cotanto amante*
> *Questi, che mai da me sia deviso*
> *La bocca mi bacio, tutto tremante.*

I wanted to say something about poetry and love. I caressed her shoulder, kneaded it with my palm, waiting for her to melt into me as she had so many times before. But unexpectedly she burst into tears. Later I realized that it was the words *che mai di mi sia deviso*—"who will never be parted from me"—that reduced her to tears. They moved her so much because she thought of us that way too. As eternally loving, never abandoned or abandoning.

Love was the only religion Hannah had held on to. If I die first, I have no doubt that she'll dress in black like the Sicilian women, mourning me for the rest of her life. I'm ashamed to admit that it gives me a moment's pleasure to think of extending my power over her, but then I feel a frisson of fear and my hands go cold. Too much, too much wild intensity. In the past it became frightening when I had to leave for any reason, to work on a film or go to a conference or read. Then she would accuse me of wanting to get away from her story.

Once I went out to meet Monica Vitti for dinner to talk about a film we were planning to do together. It was a balmy summer night and we were in Piazza Navona talking after dinner and having a cigarette. Because of the music—a jazz group was improvising and the fountains plashing—it was hard to hear. I was leaning forward, trying to tell Monica something, speaking directly into her ear, when I suddenly caught a glimpse of Hannah standing in the shadows craning her neck, trying to see more plainly. Her fists were clenched, and I thought for a moment she planned to attack.

She told me later that she felt betrayed by Monica, who was her friend as well. That she had in fact wanted to kill her, calling her every possible name: whore, piece of shit. But what enraged her most was that I was content and self-contained existing without her. It was right after that incident that I decided to take her back to her village and do a film about it and her. I also doubled my attentiveness, if such a thing were possible.

There was a story in the *Herald Tribune*—which I still read occasionally to have something to talk about with our American friends—about a woman Marine who discovered that her boyfriend had been cheating on her. Powered by rage and humiliation, she drove through the night in diapers so she wouldn't have to stop on the way. When the police pulled her over for speeding, she had rope and pepper spray, a BB gun, a two-pound drilling hammer, and pictures of bound women, making it clear she meant to kidnap and hurt her rival. How can reason even begin to understand such things? For that moment of vengeance she lost her whole life's work and her honor.

I wake up worried about this supposed memoir I am writing. I remember from before how things have to have a beginning, a middle and an end, but it doesn't mean the same thing to me now. Better T. S. Eliot's "In my end is my beginning." Would he have been willing to say that if he had been an atheist? Perhaps imagining going back into soft earth and emerging as a colorful plant. Wasn't there a legend about a woman who put her beloved's head in a pot after he'd betrayed her and she'd beheaded him, and in the spring roses grew there red as blood?

One thing is sure: everything circles back to Hannah. I started with her and I'll finish with her. Maybe a double suicide of the sort the Japanese love, the couple dressed up in wedding kimonos launched together hand in hand off a cliff, their kimonos, exquisitely painted with spring flowers, billowing so they look like giant birds in the warm air. But my liking for that is purely aesthetic. I imagine one of us will die of a weak heart and the other will climb onto the bed and take the cooling body into her arms.

I remind myself that death isn't pretty. If I had ever been tempted to see it that way, Hannah would have cured me. For years she had the most terrible nightmares about the death camps. Her most persistent one was of Mengele coming into her barracks to select the people to gas or to be experimented on, fed poisons, or submerged in freezing water and then revived. She must have been a beautiful child, but with her face filthy, standing in her ragged camp uniform, she learned to disappear.

"It was so important not to be seen, Renzo," she told me, "My life depended on it."

Even then she had a ferocious will to live. She stood looking down, her beautiful eyes hidden by dirty blond hair. Sometimes she would even rub dirt through her hair and over her skin—anything to dull the shine of her. When all her efforts to fade into the background didn't work and she was selected, she ran away and hid with her sister. But in her nightmares the barracks *capo* grabs her by her dirty neck and hands her over to Mengele.

There was a rumor among the women in her barracks that Mengele's latest project was training dogs to rape young girls. Hannah wakes screaming from a horrible dream where they are coming with the dogs to get her. Or she dreams of a friend running against the electric fence, determined to die, and she is unable to help her. The girl had given Hannah a precious gift, a wooden spoon, after hers had been stolen. Such unselfishness was rare in the camps. But it kept them from feeling like animals.

When such things have happened in real time, it is hard to "recover." Veterans of our misguided wars remind us of that, should we be tempted to forget. Hannah still jumped at sudden noises, loud sounds. But just as my memories are all jumbled up, what was confused in her was the line between nightmare and our waking life. To know what was real. Could the reality that had been so painful coexist with gentleness and warm baths, scrambled eggs and kisses?

Even after years of being here in the same house, Hannah would get lost when she went out for a walk. Our palazzo is on Vittorio Emanuele. In back, after a short section on Santo Spirito, is Via dei Banchi Nuovi, which goes into Via del Governo Vecchio then pauses at Pasquino's statue—where Gina used to post her angry rhymes about the whorishness of Rome and Berlusconi. The statue makes its square eminently recognizable. A few blocks further on is Piazza Navona, one of Rome's most famous piazzas. How is it possible to get lost there? But she does. Time after time she confuses the path there with the streets on the other side of Corso Emanuele.

There the landmark is a newspaper kiosk that you can see as soon as you open our front door. From the kiosk, if you take Banchi Vecchi to Via di Pellegrino you will end up at Campo dei Fiori and the market. She loves our Roman vegetables and fruits, especially in the summer, and must have gone to the market hundreds of times, but if she wakes up tired or is distracted by thinking of her writing, for a moment she will confuse Banchi Nuovi and Governo Vecchio with Banchi Vecchi on the other side. I have given her maps with everything marked in red and the different routes: the one to her favorite shop, the one to our friend Arianna's house, the *Campo*, and for that day or week she'll be all right but then she misplaces my map and forgets again which route is which. After years of her doing this, it began to annoy me.

"Isn't it time to let this go? To recognize how strong you are now? You're not the little girl in the camps anymore."

"Stop stop," she said putting her hands over her ears. Later she tried to explain. "Please believe me. I don't like being lost. It's just that the streets become unrecognizable. I try and remember but I can't. Oh, it's hopeless, you can't understand."

The irony, my love, is that now I do understand. I went out the other day to pick up some *cornetti* at the café on Via Giulia where we have always gone for our espressos, sitting side by side reading the *Corriere della Sera*. I took a little walk, enjoying the smell of fresh baked bread and the sight of vans unloading produce: red and green tomatoes, eggplants in their glistening purple skins, and slender green zucchini with the blossoms still intact. Then I got the idea of shopping for a birthday present for Hannah.

I crossed back over the Corso and started looking in the windows of the antique shops lining the street for a pretty pillbox to give her. I thought I would write "*ti amo sempre*" on a slip of paper and put it inside. A tower clock chimed ten. Startled, I checked my watch and, seeing that it was really getting late, turned to go home. But suddenly I'd forgotten the way. I had a memory of crossing the Corso when I left our front door but somehow that wasn't right anymore. Nothing was familiar. All the small streets seemed possible. After a few minutes of standing in one place, wondering if I should beg someone to help me, I suddenly remembered the magazine kiosk on the corner where I always crossed over the Corso in the mornings to pick up my paper before going on to the café for my cappuccino.

I didn't tell Hannah because I knew her fear for me would make her scold me. She would have made me take a map, and sketched out important landmarks. I went from near tears to laughter thinking about it—a case of the blind leading the blind. But I am touched, too, at the thought that she would try and do something so difficult for her—out of love. I determined to mark the maps myself while I still could.

When we're young we tend to think of memory as something belonging to us. There are good memories and bad ones, but aside from forgetting names occasionally, it is hard to imagine what ceasing to rely on your memory means. My mind still functions enough for me to be frightened and feel diminished. Someday, I hope not too soon, I'll cease to be alarmed; I'll slide out from under the wearisome tasks of everyday life and my poor Hannah will have to take them up.

But I'm still worrying about my failure to organize my memories into some form. At least I should put my early years with Hannah first, then Claudia, finally me, old and aging.

But that doesn't interest me now. Instead, I think of making a long list of all the dishes I cooked for her. Pasta with clams was one of her favorites, but I also made pasta Bolognese and *strozzaprete* with porcini mushrooms.

(Hannah was gleeful about the suggestion that priests were being strangled. The pope had been friendly to the Germans; even now the present pope had trouble speaking to officials of the Israeli government.) I roasted baby lamb and potatoes and baked every sort of fish in the oven: rospo, swordfish, sea bass, all roasted with tiny tomatoes. For desert I made crème caramel and hot apple torte

Another thing that frightened her was the idea she might lose her apartment. The one she had when I met her. She was paranoid about her landlady, whom she felt sure had been a

Fascist, because once when Hannah was late with the rent and had gone to hand it to her personally, Hannah had caught sight of the photo on the sideboard of a man in a Fascist uniform. It was all she could do to keep from cursing the woman, telling her how she had suffered from men like her husband and father. Instead she wrote a story. Black words leaking from her pen onto paper.

Last night there was a thunderstorm. We were lying together in our bed under the eaves when the thunder started crashing right over our heads. The eaves are so close that we have to crawl into bed on our hands and knees. I started worrying about the baby gulls on the roof below our terrace. Was the soft fluff cradling their bodies enough to keep them dry? I knew their parents—mother or father—would spread their wings as far as they could and the chicks would cuddle close. I moved under Hannah's arm and inhaled the slightly acrid but always pleasing scent, like warm grass mixed with lemon zest.

Lightning flashed blue outside. Zigzagging across the sky, punctuated by the booming of thunder. Bang bang bang.

I decided that tomorrow I would throw some bread or meat scraps down to the gulls. Our landlord, Barry, would be furious if he knew. He told our maid, Erminia, that he had poured boiling water on the eggs one year. Our terrace has a rickety iron staircase leading to a viewing platform that offers a 360 degrees view of red-tiled Roman roofs. He told her if they nested up there—they like to be able to see who's coming—to take the eggs and throw them away. Erminia had taken them and put them on the edge of our fountain. Perhaps enchanted by their color she didn't throw them out. People have a sentimental view of peasants, Liberals at least, but maybe Erminia had some other motive, something else entirely.

Erminia did have a charming naïveté sometimes. She told me that her grandfather had fought in World War II (or would it have been her father?) and in the army he had his first sight of black men. It astonished him. Once a black soldier caught him staring and asked him what he was staring at.

"I was wondering if you were a Christian," her grandfather answered.

"By 'Christian' he meant a human being like me," she explained. Erminia didn't remember what the man had answered.

In the morning I went out to look at the gulls and found them sleeping in the sun, wedged into hollows made where the tiles joined a small chimney. Their parent stood guard on the chimney top. I went into the fridge and found some leftover beef with fat I could trim. The mother gull was enchanted and doubtless will process it for the chicks.

I am in a strangely sentimental mood, wanting to see young creatures. There is a mother and baby who often come out on their terrace. They are there now, the baby all dressed up, with tiny socks and a matching hat. The mother is playing with it, tossing it up and making it laugh. She sees me looking and waves.

"*Che bel bambino,*" I call to her.

"It's a girl," she says.

"Someday you must come over and bring her for tea."

"I'd like that," she said.

She reminds me of Claudia. I think I said that Claudia attracted me because of her big breasts, but I should have added that she was nursing a child, that when she leaned near to me I could smell the sweet milk. Later, her little girl—an absolutely beautiful creature named Leila with a cascade of blond curls and big blue eyes—was part, maybe a big part, of my attraction. I liked to watch Claudia mothering and imagine how it would be to be cared for that way. My own mother wasn't able. A memory bubbles up of the fantasies I sometimes had about running my hands over Leila's body. It was so perfectly formed, so white it made my mouth water looking at her. I imagined her in the bathtub—something I saw often enough—and me kneeling beside the tub rubbing the soap over her.

"And always soap between your legs," I'd imagine myself saying, taking the soap from her and showing her how. "Or you can put the soap on your hand, like this," and I gently rub right on the rosy lips, holding myself in the other hand, out of sight.

Poor Nabokov in an early draft of *Lolita* imagined accustoming Lolita to seeing a man naked with an erection, but in that early draft she ran screaming from the house. Later he imagined her as a sly tease. But even in imagination I censored the idea of letting Leila see me. I couldn't stand the thought of frightening or repelling her. Of course, I never acted on my fantasies—jerking off fantasies, I called them to myself. I spent a lot of solo time imagining different scenarios and progressions, and sometimes when I was with Hannah, I would think of Leila when we made love.

None of this is so odd, is it? Everyone has fantasies of some sort. I would hate to think I was a pervert, a dirty old man, though I notice that somehow being old has loosened my inhibitions. I am always patting Hannah's bottom or thighs, calling her my little one, *Piccina*, even when company is here. But Hannah is an old woman like me and I'm sure the guests think it is sweet.

When Hannah takes me to the Villa Borghese Gardens near where my family lived when I was a child, we sit on the steps and I watch the young children with their nurses. The smaller children stay close. On a warm day I can see their round chubby arms and legs as they try out their steps. Their skin is so beautiful—fresh and clear, not yet written on. I drink in their freshness. Without young children there would be only bruised skin, violet and yellow unfolding like flowers on the arms of old men.

The ponies come by, led by such a man. He isn't defeated by his age. He smiles and beckons to the children. His little hat sports a red feather—it says, I am not dead yet, not yet. And the bigger children beg for a ride in his painted cart.

"Thank you for bringing me, love," I tell Hannah and she smiles at me, pats my hand, sneaks a peak at her watch. I don't begrudge her. She has things to do—her work, the house—in addition to the burden of caring for me. I consider telling her my fantasies about Leila, to see if I can get her to tell me some of hers and expose the last bits of the inner life we've hidden from each other.

"I've been reading some poetry," I say. "Nothing hard. William Carlos Williams." Nothing to harden my prick.

"I've heard the name," she says without enthusiasm.

"They are very simple," I tell her, "and you feel good after reading one. It's like eating a chocolate *Baccio*. You can savor it and carry it around like a snapshot." But right this minute I wish I'd brought something erotic—one of the Latin poets, the ones that make your loins tingle in anticipation of a good screw.

"Sounds nice," she says but I sense that she is restless, her thoughts elsewhere. "Did I tell you that Marti Restov wants to translate a couple of my poems for a new anthology?"

"No," I say, feeling suddenly tired, flaccid. "That's great." Hannah writes poetry herself. She has even been translated. She is probably better known than I am. I have a flicker of envy. But it only lasts a minute or two. I envy her much more for her intact brain.

"I've noticed that images—a white gull with pink feet, a red lily—stick better in my mind than facts or names even of people I know quite well."

"Why don't you read me something?" she says with sudden generosity. I flip through the pages of the slim volume I brought with me. "Here," I say "just a taste:"

Her body is not so white as
anemone petals nor so smooth—nor
so remote a thing. It is a field
of the wild carrot taking
the field by force.

She cocks her head and looks at me. "Anemone?"

"Five petals, red or purple or white. I love the way he makes it about degrees of whiteness and the personalities of the flowers. You're my wild carrot."

"Not sure if I should be flattered," she says.

"You should. You're no hothouse flower. You are stronger than you think."

She wraps her arms around herself and shivers as if to contradict me. I wonder what Hannah's sexual fantasies are like. I've never been rough with her, always treated her gently, trying to erase her memories of the camps, but what if she imagines pain: being tied and tormented, spanked, pinched in sensitive places? I look at her, trying to imagine myself into her head.

Later, back on our terrace, I sit in one of the intact chairs, the one with the embroidered cushion and look over my notebook. Already I am forgetting what I wrote earlier. Some of it sounds quite good. I'd be interested in it if another old man had written it.

But suddenly I see I've made a terrible error. Here I say—quite clearly in blue ink—that Hannah heard my mother playing Chopin, but Hannah didn't hear her, didn't even know her. I was confused. It's true my mother was elegant and regal. I can still remember her dressed to go out to the symphony in a blue velvet gown, her chestnut hair swept up and tamed, but Hannah didn't know her.

If Hannah had known her, would she have liked her? I think so. Funny how their meeting seems so true. Did I say that Hannah saw her dead body and kissed her face? I can't remember if I said that, but that isn't true either. I would have liked it certainly, the two women I care most about, together.

Hannah had insisted on a visit to a neurologist "just to have a baseline." I hated the idea. It suggested a progressive worsening. Before my follow-up visit I was so afraid of what the doctor would find that I threw up. My vomit was thin and green with yellow specks. An abstract painting that mesmerized me for some minutes before I got off my knees and washed my face.

It's not that my doctor is unfriendly or incompetent, but still she makes me feel as if I've dropped into a parallel universe, changing from subject to object. She scans my face, looks me over, and asks me how I'm doing. I try to be upbeat. Then she asks Hannah if she has noticed anything new since last time. Hannah tells her about my mistakes with money, my difficulty with simple arithmetic, my confusion about what things cost. My buying the seventeenth century book. I am embarrassed, like a small boy at school trying to sound out words that he doesn't know.

"I've been tired lately," I say. "I haven't been well."

The doctor exchanges a look with Hannah. I suddenly can't remember what kind of a doctor she is. Pediatrician? Geriatrician? Oncologist? I feel more and more anxious and cover it with a smile. She is talking to Hannah about some new medicines that are being tested. I protest that I don't want any medicine.

"It might help with forgetfulness," the doctor says, "brighten up your synapses. It can't hurt you." I see Hannah nodding.

"All right," I say, "I'll try it." The last thing I want is to seem unreasonable.

The doctor has pretty hands. I can imagine them stroking my face, soothing me the way you would a crying child. I read a story by F. Scott Fitzgerald once about a man, Benjamin Button was his name, who instead of growing older grows younger until he becomes a baby and floats helplessly away on a river to die. Someone made a movie of it starring Brad Pitt. Maybe I could do an Italian version some day.

Is this what is happening to me? My wish to be surrounded by children might have been a sort of foreknowing.

A wish to become a child again, like the luscious *putti* on the church ceilings with their unashamed penises and gossamer wings—fresh souls. My brief flare-up of sexual energy when I thought about Leila wasn't a sinking into prurience. It was the life force holding on before it flickers out.

The doctor isn't going to stroke my face. Instead she asks me questions. The year, the date, the place where we are now. Then she makes me touch my shoulder with my left hand while moving my right hand towards the window. I have trouble getting it. Clearly the pressure to perform is confusing me.

"I'm going to give you an address," she says finally, "and I want you to remember it while we do some other things. All right?"

I nod.

"Andrea Monte, Via Governo Vecchio, 85," the doctor says. I look at Hannah to see if this is a trick of some sort. Hannah gives me a sad little smile because that was one of the streets that she used to get lost on.

I check my mind to see if I still have the address she gave me and I do. I think of how I'm going to rattle it back at her with gentle reproof for her suspicion that I couldn't remember a simple name and address. Meanwhile she gives me some other tests, asking me to touch places on my body. To count backwards, spell backwards. "Do I have to? Do that?" I asked her. "I've always had trouble with directional things. Are all these tricks really necessary?"

"You've done very well," she says. "We're almost at the end."

Then she asked me for the name and address she had given me. It seemed to be on the tip of my tongue but I couldn't capture it even when she gave me hints or multiple choices. She says it's too early to give a firm diagnosis. The only thing that really seems to bother her is my forgetting the name and address she gave me. I try to recall it now that she's reminded me what it was and all I remember is that it was the place where my Hannah got lost. On the way home we stop at the *farmacia* and order my new medicine.

I was looking for something on my bookshelf but forgot what I was looking for. Instead a novel falls into my hands. The title is in crimson, the letters drip blood. How odd. I don't like murder mysteries except Agatha Christie's, and this author has an unknown name: Ella Erickson. Sounds Swedish. Ah, I see it's a translation and, looking at the inside flap, I see the book described as the spine-chilling story of a woman and an old man.

I begin to remember now. They'd been lovers and he'd let a gasoline lamp fall and it killed her baby. I remember thinking it was just an accident: he didn't mean to do it. But she was determined to avenge her child's death. When he became infirm and advertised for a home nurse, she took the job and set about to torture him. Ah, yes, he was becoming demented. But still able to understand how much she hates him. One day he tries to escape, tells his visiting daughter that he is being persecuted, that the "nurse" she hired isn't really a nurse but a woman who wants to destroy him.

The "nurse" pretends concern that his dementia is worsening.

"The other day," she says, "he tried to wheel his chair down to the road, yelling, 'Help! I'm a prisoner!'"

She promises to be more vigilant, not to leave him alone for a minute. He sobs in despair. I think at the end she suffocates him with a plastic bag.

A truly horrible book—though at the time I read it, I didn't identify with the old man. Now I do and it seems even more horrible. When we're sick we have to be more trusting—have to believe that the people tending us will measure out the right dose of medicine, give us the proper injections. That's why we shudder when we read in the newspapers about killer nurses who purposely inject lethal substances in their patients' veins. What could make a person do that?

Oh, come on, Renzo, you remember when your mother used to chase you around the house screaming that she wanted to kill you, enraged because you'd told a little lie or forgotten to do your addition homework. Curled up on your bed crying, rubbing your arm where she hit you, didn't you ever have murderous thoughts? No, maybe you didn't. You were too young and too vulnerable—probably just longing for her love, trying to think of ways to get it.

I think what I'm asking myself now is, when I left Hannah for Claudia, did she feel enough rage to want to hurt me? Or did she suppress it the way I did mine as a child? The way she did when the young Nazi spit on her naked body? She told me she thought of grabbing his pistol and shooting him. But her wish to live was too strong. She just bowed her head with that meek expression she had learned to put on when she was begging the guards for scraps from their pails, a piece of fruit, a peel, a rotten potato.

Love, hate, vulnerability, dependence. I write the words and make circlets of flowers around them. How hard to chart the mixtures. No recipe for love.

Sometimes I think I see the curl of her lip, a slight hint of a smile that isn't all friendly. And who is to blame her?

After I moved out all those years ago, I tried to make my absence tolerable by seeing Hannah daily and bringing her small presents when I went off on my trips. But actually my daily visits only made things worse, reminding her that I had chosen not to be with her. At one particularly unfortunate lunch—I'd come back from seeing a season's worth of new work by young German directors—she told me she had just gotten a part in a film. The director wanted her to play a Jewish woman. He thought she'd be perfect.

Did I have to tell her that the director was a nobody without any talent? I had been lecturing Hannah that she needed to be independent. Why wasn't I pleased when she made the first small steps? But I wasn't pleased. Anymore than my mother was pleased when I found a friend who invited me over to play, whose mother caressed my curls and told me what a handsome, good boy I was. That same day, over roast chicken, I criticized Hannah for not really enjoying her liberty.

"No, I don't," she said, "I hate it. It would be different if you hadn't loved me, though even then I can't imagine liking to be alone."

"You have more friends than I do. Lovers too, if you want to get down to it. It doesn't seem to stop you. And I've never objected. I'm afraid you just want me to feel guilty, to feel that I've damaged you beyond repair."

"I don't mean to make you feel bad," she said. "You haven't destroyed me—maybe made me lose a few pounds— see, I'm functioning." She moved her arms up and down like a bird ready to take off. She gave me a lopsided smile, "As for enjoying my liberty, I'm even beginning to like having the bathroom to myself."

"About time," I said. "It's been months. And you act as if I'd left you and flown off to Tahiti. I haven't vanished. You can pick up the phone anytime day or night and call me." I ground to a halt. Damn. How did she always manage to put me on the defensive? "I just can't put you at the center anymore. You've got to stop thinking of me as your grand *amor*."

"Admit it, you are repelled by me."

"Oh, sweetheart! Please don't make such a drama of it. You must know I love you. I am just trying to live honestly." She had meant to draw me close but her accusations had the opposite effect. Why did she have to insist on what wasn't there anymore? At least not in the same way. She saw I was withdrawing and turned to stone, a heavy dark basalt half-hidden in dirt. Brooding, eyebrows pulled together. I could see she wasn't listening anymore. But what should I have done? The only thing that would soften her would be to take her home, go upstairs with her, and put her to bed the way I used to in our first days together. Tucking her in, kissing her gently. But now

I sensed that wouldn't be enough. My offhand response had offended her need to be special. She was like a dog worrying a bone. She needed to consume me.

She had found a psychoanalyst who listened patiently while week after week she complained about me. He said that I was too vulnerable for the sort of love she wanted. It's true I've never had an all-consuming passion, though I was with Hannah and close to her much longer than I had been with anyone else.

Leafing through my journal to jog my short-term memory, I see that I've given the impression of devoting myself entirely to Hannah until, finally drained, I turned to Claudia. It's certainly true that I cared for Hannah, soothed and nurtured her, but I also had time for brief flings with attractive women.

I wonder if her shrink told her I am a Don Juan, one of those whose desire always outruns what a lover can give them. Does he rip away my fleecy lamb's coat and offer me up to Hannah's understanding as a ravenous wolf? Will she succumb to his view of me? I hope not. I thought of my adventures as giving me an ego massage—not to speak of a physical one. Otherwise, I couldn't have kept up as well as I did. Going to bed with someone for the first time opens up a whole new territory—a lush Edenic landscape. I was an inveterate traveler. Just like any other addict, I had to have my fix.

But it was never serious. Never before Claudia was I tempted to leave Hannah. Though several of my mistresses urged me to rid myself of her, I always succeeded in slipping away. I prided myself on remaining friends with them after I broke off, listening to their troubles, advising them. If they were really distraught, I would care for them for weeks with the devotion of a mother. I thought of myself as a trusted friend. Did Hannah know? Maybe she guessed. She certainly was always jealous. Hated my independence even when I wasn't up to anything.

I think of it as a token of my delicacy that afterwards my mistresses were always glad to have me visit. Even Claudia—who had most reason for resentment because I had broken up her marriage—said there would always be a room for me in her house. When I visited I brought candy for Leila.

But there was no way Hannah was going to settle for that back then. When she found out about Claudia, she fought tooth and nail. Then suddenly she caved in, stopped insisting on my dropping Claudia, begged me to come home.

And now finally she has me.

After I moved out, Hannah couldn't stand being alone in the apartment. She invited her older sister Leah, who lived in Israel, to come and bring her niece to stay with her awhile. She hadn't seen her for years and hadn't told her of our troubles.

At one time they had been extremely close. Leah had been with her in Auschwitz. She protected her, stole food for her, shared her plank and bedding, did more to keep Hannah alive than her mother would have done. Hannah once told me that she might have died if her mother had lived instead of being sent immediately to the gas. Her mother would have been looking desperately for a bit of candle to light on Shabbat and would have failed to see the scrap of food that Hannah needed to survive.

That had sent chills up my spine. What impressed me most was Hannah's courage in telling the truth completely, without sentiment, though she added that her mother had lost her glasses and that Hannah's last glimpse of her was moving towards the gas chamber, peering nearsightedly at the men's line for her husband and son. To me there is so much love in that image. Her mother even at the last wanting to keep her family together. At the same time, I remember that Hannah told me a neighbor offered to hide her in her cellar before the roundup of Jews but her mother wouldn't think of splitting the family up. Kept looking up at the sky and praying to the Almighty. Hannah blamed her for that.

I add *ambivalence* to my list of words defining love and draw vines around it—clinging vines.

But if Auschwitz was the mold that shaped Hannah and her sister, Leah had come out totally different. I think I've said before that her sister had become a clone of their mother. Orthodox. Totally bound up in her family. Her daughter Sarah, following the law that children must rebel against their parents' ideas, was like Hannah in many ways. She fought constantly over Israel and Zionism with her orthodox mother, replaying Hannah's own history in contemporary dress. Like Hannah, Sarah questioned everything her mother believed in. She hung out with a group of young extremists and flaunted her connection to them, accusing her mother with a sneer of being a bourgeois Fascist.

Really the only thing that Sarah and Leah agreed on was their affection for me. Without waiting to hear our story, Leah blamed Hannah for driving me away—a stance that turned Hannah livid with rage, though I couldn't help being pleased that they thought me such a treasure. Hannah's sister had always attracted me. Jet-black hair, huge dark eyes and a tendency to passionate outbursts. I wouldn't have liked to live with her extremes of emotion, but they suggested what she might be capable of in the bedroom. Leah was terrified that Hannah wouldn't have enough money to live, but Hannah explained that we would share each other's last penny if necessary but that she had decided to make a living by writing. Her sister apparently didn't take that as an economically wise choice.

Leah and Sarah had come to visit Hannah a few months after I began to live with Claudia. They shared Hannah's spare room, the library, the only one in our flowing attic space that had a door and a bathroom. I had found Hannah a lovely small apartment above a monastery garden and planned to help her with the rent, but after that terrible night-visit to my bed, I realized she couldn't be the one to move out. She had done too much moving already. No, though it hurt me to give it up, I realized she had to stay in our place.

"She obviously wanted us to get back together," Hannah told me when I called to ask how the visit was going. "She kept prodding me to see if I still loved you. And of course she saw that I did. I told her that it was you whose love was doubtful."

Relaying this to me over the phone, Hannah started to cry. All this took place months later. She had been so anguished at first that our friends would call me, frightened that she might harm herself. Gradually she became able to talk about something else when she saw them. Less like Niobe, all tears, delirious with grief. She hadn't been able to tell her sister about Claudia because she didn't want the story to turn into a narrative of "the other woman." But she also didn't want her sister to put the blame squarely on her. So she told Leah that though I seemed so amiable and caring, I had my share of neuroses, my need to be alone, for example.

Another trait Hannah's therapist might call neurotic is my own deep wish not to be blamed. I wrote her dozens of letters telling her I didn't blame her for anything and hoped she wouldn't blame me. I wrote her that, paradoxically, our happy years together were too comfortable for someone of my temperament. I pleaded with her to understand.

There was a sense in which she unmanned me, made me her pampered child. And I had a terrific sense of debt that I could never repay. It tormented me and was worst with people close to me. I found it easier to care for strangers. I couldn't be normal with her—fight and then make up—anymore than I could have been with a man whose legs had been amputated. Like the schizophrenic girl with her therapist, Hannah only felt the world was real when she was next to me, touching me, drinking me in with her eyes. Without that she wasn't really living. She felt like a sleepwalker.

But I wouldn't accept that. I kept pointing out—and making her agree with me—that she was better now than she'd been when I first moved out. She still seemed nervous but not crazy. Though sometimes I could see that, I had to believe she was better, that like Hamlet, she was only mad north-north-west and could snap out of it if she wanted to. She confessed to me how she spent time in my old closet smelling the things I had left behind. Things she had helped me shop for. Even my shit reassured her with its familiar odor. It got to the point where it was intolerable to listen to her pain. I thought making a movie about the schizophrenic girl was going to help me understand Hannah, but it just succeeded in scaring the pants off me. Madness turns out to be as elusive as love.

I can still enjoy short articles in the *Corriere Della Sera*, though my attention wanders if they have too many names of people in them. Hannah went out to get me my newspaper and espresso. I didn't feel well enough today for our café. There is a short piece about Berlusconi and a photo of him waving out the window of his black limo—his guards stationed at the four corners looking intense, brows furrowed. The newspaper has gotten some new audiotapes of him ordering prostitutes and complaining that he has to see the French president and the pope this week, so he won't have a chance to meet his mistress Francesca Pascale. He runs Italy like a Renaissance prince. If it weren't so awful, it would be funny. Sex used to be private. Now news about sex has gotten all-pervasive. Every day you hear about rapes or at least groping by highly placed politicians, even in America with the Evangelicals braying about damnation—maybe more so.

Hannah told me that there are sites on the net where they hook you up for a night, but you have to pretend that it didn't happen. If one of you begins to get attached, then it is time to move on. Hannah thinks there is a dangerous disconnect between sex and love. She can be prim sometimes but this time she may be right. People—particularly young people in our Capitalistic culture—are learning to treat each other as commodities, disposable and easily replaceable.

I look at my journal, where Hannah accused me of being repelled by her. Something about the way I described that night doesn't seem right. I treated her as abnormal, a little crazy, even psychotic. But in the beginning wasn't it that intensity that I loved? She was rightly infuriated when I told her to stop being who she was. She was totally wrapped up in me just as she'd always been, never sparing herself the danger of losing her boundaries, of not knowing where she stopped and I began. And it wasn't that she was weak. My God, how strong she must have been to survive the camps, what a sense of self! No, she opened herself, took down her defenses voluntarily. I have no right to castigate her. For a while when we were first together, I felt that all-encompassing love too. It was as though we penetrated each other's skin, breathed as one, interpenetrated, laced together. I had never had such love except maybe with my mother when I was very young, though my mother disappointed me in small ways, making me live in fear of betrayal, like the young Proust waiting for his mother's good-night kiss.

After Claudia came into my life, Hannah lived for my brief visits, always hoping that I would come back to her. I could call her anytime day or night, and she would agree to meet me rather than run the danger of not seeing me for a day or two. I might have encouraged her in words to value her separate life, but I also expected her never to say no. I could complain about how uncomfortable her total concentration on me made me feel. But obviously I liked it. I kept on meeting her, hearing every detail of her life not just for months but for years. It was bearable only when I could walk away, say I had an appointment, disappear. Otherwise it frightened me the way she asked and asked. I felt as though I'd scream if she asked me to do another thing. And when I didn't respond the way she wanted me to, she'd be overcome by a towering rage and would have to restrain herself from kicking or biting—wanting to destroy me the way she felt I destroyed her. More often she restrained herself when she was with me but wrote me long furious letters afterwards.

When finally I begged her to let me come home, I was in my late eighties. And Claudia was married to a wealthy business man. Hannah had survived a heart attack and it left her purged. I could help her, I said, help take care of her. I didn't like her being alone in that apartment. I could see that she had less need to squeeze me like an orange, getting every last spurt of juice. She even allowed herself a little contentment.

She cried, calling a cherished friend and asking if she should forgive me. The friend said, "you already have. You forgave him when you kept seeing him during the Claudia years."

Forgiving is hard.

My brother Mario came over to see me today. He is four years older—have I said that already? Sorry. When I was born, he was already a tough little kid. Mother told me he hadn't liked me from the start. She had pointed out my squalling helplessness, how I couldn't do anything, how I needed him. The only effect that had was to infuriate him, especially later when I started to crawl and knocked over his block towers. By the time I was five he had me completely under his thumb. He used to tell me frightening stories about goblins and ghouls that he said lived in the Borghese garden zoo, in cages next to the big cats, the panthers and tigers. At night one of the keepers would change into a werewolf and let them out. Our house was on the very edge of the gardens. They would be drawn by our smell, the warm blood. Suddenly my brother would stop.

"Did you hear that?" he'd ask, assuming a look of terror. "The leaves are rustling. Can't you hear them coming?" Then he would make a sound between a roar and a shriek, turn his fingers into claws, and clutch my stomach. I would invariably call for Mama who would pat my head and sigh.

"Why can't you boys get along?" She'd ask no one in particular.

"Because he's a little sissy," Mario would say and spring out the big front door, laughing ghoulishly.

So here is my brother trying to be nice to me seventy-five years later, asking how I am, what the doctors are doing. I frown at him.

His questions are perfectly innocuous but suddenly I feel consumed by rage. I hate the way he sits there with his memory intact, nothing wrong with him, hiding his smug arrogance under a fake smile. His gray eyes cool as ice. He must know, damn him, that the doctors can do very little. The only drugs around make just the tiniest difference in staving off senility. I will end up a vegetable before he finishes directing his new movie.

I try to come up with better reasons for my anger. Our father always preferred him, for one thing. He was clearly brilliant from a young age. But why did Papa have to leave him more money? Each sentence in that will stabbed me in the heart. And he didn't even know that Mario had a sick wife and two children. That might have made some sense anyway. Give to the eldest one. But we were just boys when he wrote his will. He didn't know about Hannah either, of course. Or that I'd left the only woman I really loved.

Mario comes back from the kitchen with Hannah's cookies. He offers me one. We both eat quietly and he throws the crumbs over the terrace wall. The gulls pounce, cawing like mad.

"It's rotten luck," he says. "I'm so sorry, Topo." No one has called me that—short for *topolino*—since I was a boy. I stare at him, making sure he isn't insulting me, bringing up my height—five feet, five inches—whereas he is almost six feet. Tall for an Italian.

What is the matter with me? He isn't just trying to be nice, he is genuinely sorry for me. The brother of today isn't the brother of back then. I'm the one who is stuck in the piss and mire of childhood. But my increasing incapacity makes me unjust. I want to scream. Remember me please, remember me, keep me alive in you. Somewhere. I'll just take up a tiny corner. I'll crouch very low in the corner but don't forget me.

"I can't stand the thought of life going on without me," I say. "It makes me lonely, as though I'm lying in a room full of ice, unable to move a finger while the world with its trees, birds and flowers gradually fades." He presses my hand. I can see the water welling in his eyes.

One morning when I was about ten, our cook, my mother's most trusted servant, came to me with a frightened expression.

"Your mother is still asleep," she said. "I can't seem to get her to wake up."

My mother slept in a mahogany bed with a damask canopy, like a princess, I thought. I remembered her alone, though my father slept there too, of course: the royal couple. Through one window I could see the cypresses lining our walk. Through the other, her roses. That day the gardener was planting some pansies in the border, dark violet that played against the deep reds and yellows she preferred. Around the garden were classical statues of fawns.

"Please," our cook said. "Be a good boy."

"Why can't you do it?" I asked, though I knew perfectly well that Luisa was afraid of mother, who often threw tantrums and screamed at her.

"All right," I sighed as the gardener's sheers opened beneath a fading flower. "But I don't see why you can't let her alone." Ordinarily if I frowned, Luisa would immediately soothe me, but this time she shifted unhappily from foot to foot, she wouldn't move. I was beginning to feel uneasy myself, though I didn't know why.

I don't really remember walking up to the bed. But I must have done it. Her head was on the pillow and her eyes were closed. I don't think I had ever seen her sleeping before. Her eyelids were a deep blue, almost purple. I stood and looked.

"Mother," I said, touching her lightly on her shoulder. Under her satin nightgown I could feel her warm skin. Wake up Mother, it's time." But I couldn't remember what it was time for. I shook her lightly but she wouldn't open her eyes. I don't know what made me realize that she didn't hear me, that she wouldn't wake up no matter how much I shook her or how loudly I yelled in her ear. I ran out of the room, almost bumping into Luisa who was waiting right outside. "She won't wake up," I screamed, my body hot and cold in turn. My heart was thumping like a giant frog. My knees shook so hard I could barely stand and waves of shudders passed from my head to my feet. Luisa was calling *pronto soccorso*.

When the men came with the stretcher, they took one look at her and the empty pill bottles next to her bed, scooped them up without even a word to me, and took her away.

"Someone stop them," I cried out. "They're taking my mama away."

My memory is playing tricks on me. The true horror of that scene was that I felt nothing except a mild wish not to be disturbed, a feeling that someone else should take care of this, that I was too young, too completely unready. It was wrong. It ought to be erased. But I remember no other feeling. I don't think my heart thumped anymore. No, I was preternaturally calm. A sort of blankness fell over me like a cape.

I moved and spoke but I didn't feel, not at all. I stood fascinated by her purple eyelids, but felt no curiosity—nothing but a pale cloud-like vacancy where feelings should have been. Isn't that strange? My brother was away on camping trips for prospective leaders on the Left, and before he came home I stood in front of a mirror and practiced my expressions. Horror: mouth open and distorted, eyes wide. For grief, I remembered how I felt when my dog died. Then my motions had been perfectly natural. I sobbed and tossed my head. I begged to dig his grave myself and carried him to it, wrapped in a blanket. Now I screwed up my face and tried to force tears from my eyes, but they stayed dry. I felt nothing at all.

I was afraid that my brother would notice—that I would somehow be excommunicated. He would point out my heart-lessness. In fact, if my friends had called and invited me to a party, I would have gone. Laughed and joked, eaten until my stomach hurt. But Mario was wrapped up in his own feelings, unless like me he was numb. I never asked him, and we never spoke of it.

Last night I wandered for hours in different landscapes. One was a ruined city. You could tell it had once been beauti-ful from the arches still standing, entrances now to nowhere. One arch had signs of fire along the top. The stones were blackened. I stood at the entrance wondering if I should walk through it. There were so many arched entrances I was afraid I'd get lost. Perhaps if I counted. I'd go in the third. I turned around and tried to memorize the arch I was going through but it was just like all the others. I'd have to remember it was the third from where I was standing. I had no pencil or paper the way I do now to write down the things I know I'll forget. I have pads, I have different color pens—they are scattered everywhere in our apartment. This morning I found one behind the classical statue of an athlete near our bed. Another in our little kitchen alcove next to the salad twirler. But in my dream I had nothing to help me. Nothing and no one. Still, something propelled me. It turned out there was a whole city alive in the ruins—scavengers and homeless men lying in their tattered blankets against the walls, worn boots on their feet or under their heads.

I remember how Hannah had told me about the impor-tance of boots in the camps. If someone's boots were stolen they'd probably die. They made every effort to hold them together—with bits of string, or if they had holes they'd stuff them with paper. In our brutal world today, people more than ever need their boots.

Hannah told me that during the long march through Germany at the end of the war, her boots fell apart and she walked barefoot, her feet infected and full of pus. And no one in the villages threw them bread. She tried hard not to return their hate but couldn't accustom herself even to the sound of German. It made her sick.

In my dream I was suddenly afraid someone would rob me. Still, I counted to three and went under the third arch into a narrow street. I tiptoed past the sleepers. Then the scene changed and I recognized the landscape with its vine-covered hills. I was in a green field near our tower—part of an old palazzo outside of Todi. I knew if I got there I'd be safe. Our family had owned it for generations. It had protected the peasants from marauders in the Middle Ages. We even have a heraldic device, a lion *couchant* with crossed spears. I moved towards it but was immediately lost in tall grass. A woman's voice suggested I turn left, but I was too afraid. Grass was everywhere, mounded into shapes like freshly dug graves. There was no clear trail. An animal appeared, a bobcat, lean and sinuous. I threw it some bread to keep it away, but instead it came towards me, its eyes glinting red. I woke, heart pumping.

I fell back to sleep almost at once, but no sooner was I asleep than I had another dream. In this one, I was being slowly pushed towards a well. I tottered on the stone edge. Terrified, I awoke and called out for Hannah. "Hannah, Hannah," I said in a strangled voice, "I fell into a well. I was covered in mud. In my eyes, in my mouth, everywhere." She took me in her arms and comforted me, shushing me like a child, rocking me against her breasts. "It was just a dream," she said with a hint of severity. She hates it when I talk about a dream as if it were real. She doesn't understand how real it is for me, wandering like Alice, changing my size and shape. Powerless.

Our bed is just a platform set under the eves in our *attico*, where the one sleeping on the inside will bang his head if he get up too quickly. The ceiling there is that low. I can't remember the right word for the protrusion with a window at one end. Starts with a *g* I think—*goal, ghost, growl, ground.* Ah yes, *gable.* I'm not much of a carpenter but this bed was one of my most successful achievements. Since we both read a lot before going to sleep, I screwed two small lamps onto the gable's sides.

When we were first married, we used to sit there, cozy as birds in a nest. And since our backs were to the window, I put a mirror on the frame so we could see a reflection of the view behind us. The window holds a splendid view of the *Gianiculo.* The dark green forests marching up the hills, the ancient walls, and the papal palace at the top. After I moved back to our beloved apartment in Rome, when my prostate weakened and I had to get up several times in the night to pee, we turned the bed sideways with me on the outside with a clear route to the hall and the bathroom. But now—whether it's been weeks or months I'm not sure—since I walk in my sleep, Hannah moved me to the inside where she will notice if I try to move.

I used to find our maid Erminia staring at the mirror suspiciously. I'm sure she thought it was there for nefarious purposes—to reflect the tangle of our naked bodies when we made love. Alas, I can't do that much anymore. Now at most she holds it and squeezes gently. Is it an act of charity, I wonder? If I try to enter, it goes soft. But still, it is sweet.

"Go to sleep now," she repeats.

"I'll try." I say, but I know I won't be able to. My nightmare images merge with hers. I think of the way she lived at Auschwitz and how even when she was dropping with fatigue she had to be aware of what was going on around her—someone being suffocated in her bed for her rations, or her boots. Alert to the approach of danger, I can't imagine what she went through though for years. I've tried to, tried to depict parts of her experience in my films. But I always stopped before the gates to Auschwitz—there is a region that shouldn't be touched. It would invite participation in the Nazi crimes—sadomasochism, even pornography—inviting us to peer with the guard through the small window into the showers where people were being gassed. The only thing Hannah would let me film was her life "before," in an impoverished Romanian village that would have been of little interest if we didn't inevitably imagine the box cars waiting with their open doors.

In those transports, people died every day. I'm sure I would have gotten a cough or a stomach ailment—shit out my insides. I was always something of a sissy. Even when I had a headache or a bad tooth I was afraid, complained, needed to be tended. My only danger now is my failing brain. Looking up at the huge worm-eaten beams above my head, I wonder if my dreams are messages. Watch out, they are telling me, you are about to fall. Notice how you shuffle off balance when you walk, almost falling when you hit a tiny crack in the pavement. The well, the mud, show me where it will end. All my efforts to remain alert, to be vigilant—will fail.

What matters to me now are the things that nourish love, the rest is the victory of stone and the enemy and death—the victory of stone and the mud and the terrible ground.

Hannah enrolled me in a film club of some sort and I started going through some of the films that inspired me in my early days when I was still an assistant director, when Fellini's masterpieces *La Strada* and *Le Notti di Cabiria* exploded like bombshells. I still thought of myself as a Communist but I had something of a double standard. Communist in politics, but never able to stand doctrinal art. I found it exhilarating that film didn't have to be only about social problems. Fellini kept some of the best of neo-realism's heritage, the sincerity and belief in humanistic values, but his own vision was metaphorical, mysterious, poetic. *La Strada* was about an inner journey. Its ending so profound you couldn't put it into words. I played it over and over, each time seeing new things. It makes me happy that I still can feel its power. It even infuses me with a temporary strength. Every time I get to the part where Giulietta Masina, running away from the circus, stops to examine a bug—she has a curious enigmatic smile—I start to cry. I know what is coming. As if by magic a troop of musicians appears and she follows them into town where a religious ceremony is taking place. It is a mysterious event that suggests her faith in life and makes her a sort of secular saint. Masina was Fellini's wife, of course. I wonder whether the circus strongman's complete inability to understand and value her character related to Fellini's marriage. He places her next to a circus strongman, a brutal and unsympathetic character. But Fellini allows even this creature a moment of truth when he cries at the end, after she dies. He finally understands her worth.

I am circling around a subject that frightens me. How to die without faith. Isn't it the main role of religion to help us accept our mortality? Going on to a better place with a loving father and, if you are a Catholic, a Virgin Mother who will always plead your case with the supreme authority. It sounds boring, frankly.

I want, need, long for the love of people here, of my Hannah.

We are having a weekend in the country. I am in the living room on the small sofa that was in Mother's room in Todi, with the fur rug over my knees. Hannah comes up from the rustic kitchen with a glass of juice. She won't let me drink wine anymore because it makes my memory worse. That's a real loss. She sits next to me and snuggles close to make it up to me. We are watching *La Strada*. After a while the film's words tire me and I turn the sound down low, but I still get pleasure from the images, especially the ever-changing expressions on Masina's face. I like to think I'd have recognized the love there, seen how special it was. I put my arm around Hannah and pat her hip, my favorite part of her. It's as though all her womanliness resides there.

"Do you remember my film, *Night in Florence*?" I ask her.

"Of course," she says, "I like it very much. It's so sensual. Beautiful." She tugs her braid, brushing it absentmindedly against her neck. I always used to untie it myself and spread her hair over her shoulders before we made love.

The film, one of my first solo efforts as a director, was about a young Jewish woman engaged to a famous professor whom she had admired for his intellect. For their honeymoon he takes her to Florence and she falls in love with the statue of David in the main square. She realizes that all the professor's descriptions of Michelangelo's life and the making of this statue aren't worth the passion she feels looking at the curves of David's buttocks, his sex, his slim ankles, his curls. After they spend an excruciating day touring other masterpieces, the professor announces, as though he is conferring a huge favor, that he wants her to work for him typing and taking notes—he is writing on the Italian Renaissance. That night she packs her bag and runs away with the desk clerk, a man with a handsome profile and no English.

"I've always liked it too," I say wistfully. "I wish I'd had the courage to continue with more like that instead of those social comedies that I can't even bear to watch now."

"The audiences liked them," she says with an ambiguous smile.

She caresses my cheek. She gave up her reluctance to write about Auschwitz several books ago and became known as a witness. A critic once referred to her work as a sort of sacred text no more open to criticism than the Bible. Her last book though—and I don't know why I haven't mentioned this—was about us, her and me. In it, she saw her love as a "splendid disaster," but one she would always cherish. I am proud of her, of course, but though I always urged her not to spare my feelings, the portrait she paints of me isn't flattering. And no one would think of treating my work as sacred text. Feeling under-appreciated tires me out. Why brood? In a few years I'll be dead and my films forgotten. That's the trouble with Art—you're either someone or no one…or at most a minor someone.

Back in Rome, while Hannah waters the plants on the terrace, I try to catch up with time. It moves so fast these days, I'm flooded with memories. My life with Hannah—Hannah herself—has returned to what it/she was at the beginning. My sense of time is confused. The sun catches Hannah's hair as she moves and I remember the glorious gold it used to be. Now I can't remember ever seeing it turn.

When I was young my pony had the most magnificent mane flowing down over his withers. It glinted gold like Hannah's hair when I rode under the cypresses over to the arena. No, the arena I am remembering wasn't at our country place, it was in Rome where every spring they had the big horse show, and riders from all over the world would come. I didn't ride in the show but I had lessons in the arena wearing my new jodhpurs and my tweed jacket. My boots shone like mirrors. My teacher was an old German, very strict, who used at shake his whip at me when my knees weren't tight enough or my shoulders sagged or I lost a stirrup going over the jump.

I wish I was still able to ride. There was something wonderful about the closeness, the warmth of affection when my pony greeted me with a soft whinny, nuzzling in my hand for sugar or a carrot. Then adjusting my body to the gait, the languorous slowness at a walk, drinking in whatever is growing, buzzing, singing—feeling the seasonal fog, the heat of the sun, the light, moist air.

Hannah used to tease me, saying that my sympathy for the liberal democrats would last just as long as I wasn't caught in a traffic jam next to tens of blaring radios. But still, my summers as a child in Todi playing with the peasant children did give me a genuine sympathy and liking for them and a whole range of others who were close to the land. And later, it was part of Hannah's attraction. My tutor put an end to my play with the village children when I was about eleven. Hannah brought them back to me. Her frankness and strength, the will that got her through the camps were qualities I had seen in the village children. They weren't coddled when they were sick; they were strong-bodied, clever at all the things that kept them alive: carding wool, cutting hay, swimming in icy water to save a younger comrade who had slipped off the bank. Hannah tells me I idealize them—though in her village stories she does too.

What a difference from the dancing classes in Rome. There the little girls all wore taffeta dresses and white gloves, their glossy curls drawn back. My little girlfriend in Todi wore patched skirts and ran barefoot through the fields. She was especially bold. We wrestled in the new hay, and once she kissed me. I used to come and watch her milk their family cow. I would beg her to let me try. Her father would beat her if she did, she said. She pretended to be angry with me and would squirt warm milk into my face. Later I borrowed my brother's bike for her, and we would bump along the dirt roads, occasionally stopping to steal some fruit from our neighbor's trees.

I was out for a walk with Hannah just now and we ran into my old friend Peter. He is in charge of all the dubbing of foreign films, and his studio is ten minutes from us on Via Margutta. He came up and hugged Hannah and then me. Usually she would have called out a name: "Oh, Pete, how good to see you," but for some reason she didn't. I was looking at his face. I knew I knew him, but I just couldn't remember who he was. Not just his name and his profession but also his wife's and children's names were lost. I hoped it didn't show in my face but I am afraid it did. If I had seen him in his studio I think it would have come to me, but on the street like that....

After what seemed like an eternity Hannah asked about his wife, Linda, and his name came back to me: Peter. I was so frightened that I couldn't stop trembling and had to take a hot bath when we got back home. While I was soaking, I looked up at the clock on the wall—an antique that had belonged to my grandfather—and had trouble reading the time. Wasn't sure if I was looking at the big hand or the little one. Which one told the hour? I wasn't sure, and as I tried to figure it out I remembered that at dinner at Othello's last night I couldn't figure out the tip and, worse than that, I couldn't add it to the main part of the bill. I seem to have forgotten arithmetic. No, I won't say that. I just need to concentrate.

No more leaving it to my automatic pilot. I may even get a brain gym. If you practice the exercises on your computer regularly, they say your memory can improve dramatically—if you're lucky that is. Or maybe I should just get together a file of small photos of close friends with their names and professions: a small dictionary of the people who matter. For the others in a more distant circle it will be enough to say, "Forgive me I'm blocking your name...a senior moment."

We'll both laugh. Inside, of course, I won't be laughing.

I've been thinking a lot about artists who have been battered by the world but still managed to create, like Munch or Van Gogh. Sometimes the strain was too great. You'd think that having created even one jewel such as the church of Sant' Ivo, Borromini would have felt safe, embodied forever in stone that seemed to dance around you as you stood inside. But he not only killed himself, he did it painfully, punishingly. Perhaps he thought of it as art, the sword he used, a ceremonial blade that would have pleased a Samurai warrior. Of course there is the art of living too, and man must choose, as Yeats so eloquently pointed out, perfection of the life or of the work. A blade in the gut perfects neither one.

Yeats insisted on keeping his journals natural, not honing them or imposing a structure, just following his thoughts.

He insisted on not even linking them for fear of surrendering to literature, when what he wanted was casual thoughts, an expression of his life. Isn't that what I want too? Whatever life is left to me.

Yesterday, Hannah brought home a new biography of the great painter Arshile Gorky, written by an Armenian compatriot of his. I wasn't up to doing more than flipping through it, but I got the impression that the author was making an elaborate plea for the importance of Gorky's Armenian heritage. Funny how when he was alive and poor his American patrons—friends of my friend Lucian—had to beg the museums to take a painting as a gift. Can you believe that in his lifetime only nine paintings were sold! And now that he's dead everyone wants to claim him. Poor man. But God, the paintings are beautiful. And after his last show, when that self-important critic Clement Greenberg gave him suggestions for improving his technique, only one sold. No wonder he was depressed. How would I fare with a colostomy? A broken neck, a prostate operation, my work destroyed in a fire? Badly, I think, though no one knows ahead of time just how much he can stand before he breaks. Perhaps the worst thing was that Gorky's wife retreated to her parents' home in Maine when he was at his worst, leaving him with his despair.

I came here to help Hannah after her heart attack but now I'd be lost without her. Lost. Dead in a month.

Towards the end Gorky needed his wife—Mougouch, as he called her—to be with him around the clock. If she was gone even for an hour his anxiety would drive him to the point of insanity. I shudder reading this. I sometimes have anxiety attacks in the middle of the night, but they can be quelled by moving closer to Hannah, sniffing her, reassured by the warmth radiating from her skin like a young animal. If she was out and I wasn't sure she'd come back, how excruciating that would be. Even if she is five minutes late coming back from a lunch date, I have to struggle with my fears. What if she's had another heart attack and is even now being rushed by ambulance to the hospital? I can soothe that worry by remembering she has a cell phone with my number. Someone would call me. But what if I had cause to think that she was meeting another man, someone I knew well? Luckily we are old and even at my worst I can't imagine it, but Gorky was still young, and his wife was very beautiful. Besides, hadn't she told him about her weekend with Matta?

My mother didn't have betrayal as an excuse. My father adored her. But that's the thing about losing control of your thoughts. They proliferate inside your skull, sending out tendrils everywhere. Time changes into something murky, like mud. You have to swim through muck and you can't, and no one is there to help you so you load your pockets with stones and go down to the river.

I don't think that could ever happen to me. I've been inoculated against suicide. But other things frighten me. Becoming a fool, a Punch in a Punch-and-Judy show. At the gym under the Spanish steps—Hannah arranged for a taxi to pick me up twice a week—something upsetting happened. There was another old man who was mumbling to himself as he dressed. I couldn't really make out what he was saying but I was struck by his clothes. They looked like Armani sport clothes. Very trendy and too tight for his thighs. He could barely squeeze into them. A few minutes after he left, they made an announcement asking people to cover up, and soon his wife came into the locker room to search for his clothes because in the early stages of a memory disease, he had taken someone else's. His wife was mortified and could hardly hold her head up. You know how important the *bella figura* is in Italy.

I would hate for Hannah to be humiliated by my behavior if I start to lose it. I see old people on the street sometimes, laughing or singing, happily freed of their inhibitions. There are stories about an uncle of mine who moved to New York with his family, running away from his Park Avenue apartment and skipping down the street. He always ended up at Bloomingdale's bargain basement, happily stroking the fabrics on the ladies' lingerie table.

The days before he died, Gorky was manic. He walked the streets in Greenwich Village, yowling, calling friends out of bed to help him escape his loneliness. A few months before that, he'd broken his collarbone and fractured two vertebrae in a horrific car accident. The treatment involved painful traction—foretelling the noose? He told the nurse that he felt like an onion peeled down to the core. Feeling even the trembling of a leaf. His wife wrote to Wolf and Ethel Schwabacher, Gorky's most devoted patrons, saying he needed a place to live that was his own. The uncertainty about his wife was killing him.

Somehow as I was reading, I felt tears trickling down my face. I wiped them away but more came. Gorky was so afraid. He needed a home as much as he needed his wife. I was suddenly transported back to our house in Rome in the gardens of the Villa Borghese. The ambulance men dressed in blue smocks were carrying my mother away on a stretcher.

"Quickly. *Fai presto*," I heard one say: "hurry." For some reason he was carrying an axe.

I sat with my brother on the piano bench and watched as though it were happening to someone else. The way you'd look at a movie. Inside me nothing moved. It was too unbelievable to take in.

Later, I heard them talking in the villa's kitchen, the cook and someone else talking about who might take me in if my mother died.

My tears come faster and I put my fingers up to feel them, hot against my hands. I remember now how I stood trembling beside her hospital bed. Was it the hospital on Via Ripetta? Or San Giovanni? No, that's where they took Hannah after her heart attack. When she couldn't talk for almost a week. She hardly speaks of it but I know she never likes to be far away from help. I don't know where they took my mother, but I remember now how I stood beside her bed in intensive care and begged her to wake up.

"Please. I need you," I said. "Please." There were tubes in her everywhere.

I go on reading about Gorky. How he was almost insane with rage at his wife for betraying him with Matta, for leaving him just when he needed her most. He called his friends one by one, hinting that he was going to do something, asking obscurely for help.

His friends waited too long, his biographer tells us, they strolled through the house looking for him. Seeing a rope in the barn and another in the garden. Finally, hearing a dog bark, they found him in a shed hanging from a rafter, his neck free of the brace. His feet almost touching the floor. A foot away he had written a few words with white chalk. "Goodbye, my loves." Amazing: I never cry, but now I cry harder, as though all the tears stored up since my boyhood are pouring out.

"I need you," I heard myself saying to my mother. How could you do this when I was so young? How could you force me to witness you with your bruised eyelids like wilted violets shutting you away from me. I had forgotten until now that one fearful moment when I touched the oxygen tube, so angry that I was tempted to pull off all the wires.

The nurse who had been watching me came nearer.

"Best not to touch your mother now," she said putting her hand on my shoulder.

I guess after that I went dead inside. I certainly stopped crying. I didn't cry at the funeral, still angry, wanting to punish her by my stony silence.

The sunset tonight took me by surprise. It turned the sky into a furnace, a refining fire of orange and rose banded by purple clouds. It offered me something delicious, like a mother offering a taste of some special food to a child—raspberry ice, or coffee-colored caramel, or toffee. Suddenly I remember how my mother sometimes set up taffy pulls for my birthday. Because my brother and I were both Leos, she insisted we share a party. It annoyed him to have my friends and me in the same space, but I was in heaven.

I remember when I was showing off to a little girlfriend, I grabbed the taffy while it was still hot and scorched my fingers. I didn't stop though and we—her name was Chiara—pulled and pulled, twisting it into fanciful shapes as it got thinner and lighter. Unlike the sunset colors, it didn't disappear. It made good on its promise, only melting away when it was safely in my mouth. Looking back, I am struck by how normal Mother looked, just like other mothers I knew, and so beautiful in her hat with the violets. But I'm not complaining. I'm glad to have the image of her laughing and licking her fingers. It's as if the horrible images of her unconscious in the hospital slipped aside for an instant and let it through.

Hannah got me an audio book. I've never listened to books on tape, so this is new to me. At first the voice doesn't seem quite right for the words, but after a while I get used to it. Hannah chose the book on a whim because of the title: *Crying at the Movies*. The book about the author's experience of the death of her father. She had not cried when he drowned or at the funeral or afterwards. Then suddenly one day she found herself crying at a movie—*House of Cards*—where a character experiences a loss but can't speak about it. The book was eloquently written, no doubt about it, and the force of the voice magnified the effect. But after a while I began to be angry with the author for her self-indulgence. I mean, she certainly wasn't alone in losing a parent at a young age and having no one to talk to about it.

"Other people have fits of depression, too," I say to the voice on the audio book. "Don't take yourself so seriously. Moods go up and down."

I laugh a bitter cackle. Fine thing for me to be telling someone else to perk up. I turn off the audio and go to the kitchen, looking for Hannah. I peer at her dolefully, feeling as if a black hole is expanding inside me, sucking the colors of life away. I can see at a glance that she is preoccupied, probably over that rift with the director who wanted to do a treatment of her last book—the one about the young survivor whose cousin, sent to welcome her into their family, initiates a torrid romance by raping her! I think it is one of her most powerful, cutting close to the bone. In any case, she's in no mood to baby me and I don't blame her. I think I am becoming younger every day now, like Benjamin Button. It's hard even to remember how I cared for Hannah in the early days, comforted her, taught her, surrounded her with love.

I feel myself diminishing more and more now. It makes me want to feel whatever pain I've shoved down and put out of sight. I'll never be like Hannah, who insists that life is sweet, but at least I'll have experienced my despair before I give it up and just go around giggling at my own foolish jokes and patting the mink coats of ladies at the opera.

What grieves me most is that my body is turning against itself. My eyes, once bright instruments of seduction, are inflamed and tired. They need to be moisturized and heated to bring back circulation. Soon there will be no circulation. The cells of my gums are turning against each other. Instead of eating other creatures, they are eating their brothers. Even my teeth are being hollowed out from within. My gut gives me constant low-level signals of distress. My prostate doesn't bear thinking about.

"You know darling, you are getting to be a bit of a bore," Hannah says.

"It's mortality. Just think how awful it would be if people lived forever."

A terrible thing has happened. Our neighbor's brother and sister-in-law have been killed in a car accident, leaving a seven-year-old boy. There are no other relatives—both sets of grandparents are dead, so our neighbor, whose name escapes me at the moment, has taken him in. When I was on the terrace throwing some bread crumbs to the gulls—Italian baguettes don't crumble well, they're too crusty—I sensed movement on the adjoining terrace and saw a little face, lit by extraordinarily blue eyes, peering through the lattice separating our terraces.

"Would you like to come visit and help me feed the seagulls?" I asked him. He nodded, mute, and I unlocked the lattice gate. Something about his face as he ran to look over the terrace wall at the gulls reminded me of Giulietta Masina when she studies the bug on a leaf by the road after she has lost everything. His face was begging to be surprised by life.

"I have a new mommy now," he says, as though it is the most natural thing in the world.

"Maybe you should have asked her if it was okay to come over," I say, half to myself. He shakes his head. "She said it would be good for me to go outside and get some sun. Sunshine has a lot of vitamins in it. It's not like going into a bathroom."

I must have looked puzzled because he added. "You can only go with a relative, boys with boys, girls with girls. It's a very important rule." He had a book tucked under his arm and he leaned down and put it carefully on the wooden table next to the sofa. It was an Italian translation of one of the *Oz* books. Then he looked at me to see if it was all right to stand on the sofa. It had big white cushions. "Don't worry. It's all washable," I told him. He had to stand on the sofa bench to see over the terrace wall.

I am always frightened when children get near the edge of things. Imagining cliffs crumbling or little bodies slipping between guard rails. Maybe in the end that's why I didn't have children. With my anxieties and Hannah's memories of unspeakable violence, our child would have been a nervous wreck.

The roof where the gulls are practicing for flight is about fifteen feet below us and it's slanted, so if you fell you'd probably roll right off onto Corso Vittorio. Sometimes the wind takes the young birds near the edge.

"What's your name?" I ask him.

"Roberto," he says. I put my arm around his waist, taking no chances on his losing his balance, with the other hand I give him some bread and table scraps. "Don't throw it all at once" I tell him but he isn't listening and is clearly enjoying himself. He really is the most beautiful child, with his golden hair and rosebud mouth.

"Where do they go when it rains?" he asks. The three small birds are huddled together next to the chimney where one of their parents stands guard.

"You see those tiles down there, next to the wall with what looks like hay or straw next to it? They cuddle up there. When they were smaller they slept under their mother's wing."

I stopped. Why did I have to bring up mothers? It seemed like the idea was on the tip of my tongue, ready to roll off. He didn't say anything but I'm sure he was thinking: what if they didn't have a mother? I felt a moment's anger at the young *signora* next door. Why didn't she invite the boy to do something with her? Was he just supposed to sit outside and sun himself or play jacks with the little ball I saw in his pocket? Ah well, she had her baby to think of.

I went in to get some more bread and we continued in companionable silence. After we finished he noticed some tiny red spiders running along his arm.

"They won't hurt you," I told him, but he was methodically squashing them. They left tiny points of red on his jacket. He looked up at me to see if I approved. I grunted, softly noncommittal. "They are a bit of a nuisance," I said.

Were I a Kleinian psychoanalyst, I'd have asked him if he was imagining the crash that killed his parents, expressing his anger, or covering himself with blood-like stains, participating in their fate. But he didn't need to tell me that or anything else. Several of the red spiders were crawling up his leg. He was wearing shorts and his leg was very white and shapely. I thought of Thomas's Mann's hero, Gustav Von Aschenbach, in *Death in Venice,* and how he is completely undone by a boy's beauty. In my case, seeing the boy's youthful beauty doesn't make me want to disguise my age by dying my white hair black and patting my face with makeup, and of course I know there is a vast difference between a boy of six or seven and an adolescent. Just as there is a vast difference between a man in his fifties, like Mann's hero, and a man of eighty-eight like me.

Roberto tires of squashing spiders and goes over to look at the wall fountain. "May I turn it on?" he asks, and when I show him the switch, he pulls it with pleasure and then holds his hands in the flow, rinsing them clean. Soon after that his new mommy calls him for *merènda,* the mid-morning snack, and I am left thinking of what he has given me in that short time. For at least an hour I have felt not young but ageless, my body simply a container, a shell that enables my "me" to interact with beauty. Nothing hurt me while the boy was here. Is pleasure the best antidote for pain? I'll have to make a list of pleasurable things. See more art shows, cuddle more with Hannah. But mainly I think there needs to be a change in attitude, though I'm not sure exactly what that implies. Perhaps a coming to terms with death. I look at a small white flower in the pot that Erminia brought me from the country. When I sit very quietly looking at it, the petals seem to exude a milky light.

Some time after that, I am sitting on the terrace, trying out the new eye drops my doctor has given me. Artificial tears. "It saves me the trouble of crying," I tell Hannah. But really my eyes feel a lot better. I like to look over the terrace wall into the windows of all the apartments gathered around the palazzo's stone courtyard. I also look at the terraces to see how their roof gardens are doing. Ours is by far the most beautiful with its olive tree, ferns, cacti, and oleander, with purple passionflowers climbing on strings above the doorway, making a shaded place when the sun is too strong. My favorite roof garden is at our level and every morning around nine, a woman comes out to it and takes the hood off a canary cage, and the canary, a splash of lemon yellow, bursts into glorious song.

At the same time, I hear the boy's high-pitched voice on the next terrace and, peering through the lattice, I can see his head moving along under the laundry hung up to dry. He is talking to the young *signora*, his voice full of polite respect for the grown-up. After a minute or so, he puts his head against the lattice.

"I have to go out now for a while," he says. "I'm going to help with the shopping and maybe get a treat."

I am amazed by the disappointment I feel that I can't have him right away. If I had ever had a child, I would have had a grandchild like this boy. I remember when my friends, when we were in our sixties, all together as if they've been choreographed, switched from talking about their children to talking about their grandchildren. Their delight seems to stem partly from being able to enjoy them without responsibility. Without anxiety, everything the baby does is exciting, promising. Maybe that's how I have to learn to think about getting old; I have to find what is going on in my body and mind interesting, but at a distance. Like a Buddhist.

I do wish though that people could maintain their looks the way Hannah's big black cat Mignon does. Her fur is still full and glossy. She moves a little stiffly, but there is nothing that is visibly disfigured like my arthritic hands, all gnarled and twisted.

The next afternoon his "mother" lets him come to me for the afternoon *merènda*. I told her we had just received a fresh honeycomb from Todi, from our bees there. Our caretaker had something to do in Rome and brought it with him. I took Roberto into our tiny kitchen.

"It's so small," he said and I explained that we used to eat out a lot. He nods politely and carries his plate out to the terrace. Honey is dripping down his face. I tie a napkin around his neck.

"When I was small I used to get a net for my head and then I could go with our caretaker to watch him smoke the bees and take out the frames full of honey from the hive."

"Does it hurt them, the bees?"

"No, they'll come back after a while and make more. It's just to keep from getting bites."

"I had a bite once," he said, "and my mommy put mud on it…my real mommy." Then he sat quietly.

This is the kind of quiet that lasts a lifetime.

"They are buried in the English cemetery. My mother was English. I saw their grave," he adds. "It is under a tree, big as this." He held his arms wide. "It's at the very edge of the cemetery next to the wall. Soon there won't be any more room for new graves and then people will have to stop dying." He gave a strangled laugh and was quiet again.

Were they really buried there? I wondered. I thought you had to be famous. Like Keats with the obituary he wrote for himself. *Here lies one whose name was writ in water* is etched on the chaste stone that gives you a pang every time you look at it.

"Would you like me to read to you?" I asked him after a couple of minutes. He was frowning slightly and I thought I saw the beginning of tears. He had his book with him in a little sack. He sat down next to me on the white sofa, and I began to read about Dorothy and Ozma and the wicked Nome King. I wonder if he has picked this story because of the family turned to stone—no, to glass or porcelain—by the Nome.

As if reading my mind, Roberto put his hand on my biceps. "You have a strong muscle," he said hopefully.

"I used to," I said. "But now—I know some magic tricks, tricks with cards. Maybe some day I'll show you."

Some days are worse than others. Following my own advice to cuddle more, I try when I wake up early to hug Hannah and lie next to her, spoon fashion. But she says it keeps her from getting back to sleep and rolls away from me with a perfunctory pat. I groan. She pays no attention.

What if she tires of me and my sagging flesh? No, after all these years I don't think she will. But perhaps I should encourage her to go out more and see friends. Still, she has her work and there she is at her typewriter—old as Methuselah—writing yet another book of witness. I wonder if I am using too much of her life in my scribbles here. I once told her she could say anything she wanted about me. What did she say then? Probably only "Thank you." She knew from the beginning she would write what she wanted.

When Hannah reminded me that our friend Lucian's funeral was at four this afternoon, I got an awful headache. Somehow I had managed to forget that he died. Then when she told me, for a minute I thought it was my mother's funeral she was talking about. My brother said our mother had a better funeral than she deserved. Friends appeared who hadn't seen her in years: the daughter of a famous judge, artists, members of the Senate and friends of my doctor father paid their respects. Father had been in the Senate, too, working on Liberal health bills. He would have been in favor of the vaccine to protect young girls from sexually transmitted disease that caused such an uproar here when it was first introduced. Senators beat their breasts and poured out eloquence against the idea of such things in a Catholic country. Are these children going to have intercourse? Are we encouraging schoolchildren to have sex?

I'm unable now to get as far as the toilet, and I throw up in the sink. After three bouts it got plugged up and Hannah had to call Erminia's husband to clear it—the same man who fixed the big pot on the terrace when it blew over in the storm. He's really a mason but doesn't mind doing our odd jobs.

When he came, he was very kind and suggested chamomile tea. That made me feel like a child again. My peasant nurse used to prescribe that too—I never liked it. I must have been a difficult child. Getting sick was one of the ways I used to get attention. Or at least I tried, but my mother couldn't be lured to my bedside, she had a horror of germs and would never come near me. If I seemed seriously ill, say with bronchitis, she'd hire a nurse. I remember one of them wore a stiff white uniform and put mustard plasters on my chest. I cried and cried but my mother never came.

Even after the vomiting subsided I kept getting surges of stomach acid in my throat. I told Hannah I didn't think I was up to going to the funeral. She looked at me with that slight curl of the lip that expresses a suppressed criticism and offered me a panoply of pills. The standard one—what is it, *Lomatil?* And charcoal, which usually worked but this time did not. Hannah was angry.

"You know you have to go anyway," she said finally, stating the obvious.

"Well, he won't know will he?" I said. "And it's not like I have a Nazi *capo* counting me present for a work detail."

Then I apologized. That was a terrible thing to say—or maybe I just thought it. I hate it when I don't live up to my view of myself as empathetic, warm, and caring. But right now I was having trouble feeling anything but my gut.

"Of course, I'll go," I said. "Poor old Lucian. Life had become a burden to him." He was one of the last friends from my younger days. "How could I even think of not going?"

Hannah hugged me and went to look in my closet for my dark suit and a proper shirt. I pushed her aside and found them myself. I was always something of a dandy, a smart dresser, though recently I'd downgraded to khakis and blue work shirts. The only sign of my former self is that they're tailor-made.

I remember going to a jazz club with Lucian and his wife, Gabriella. Lucian used to be an attractive man. He had a slew of girlfriends before he settled down with her. It's hard to believe he is gone, vanished from the earth. No, not vanished but about to be reabsorbed; he'll be held down by shovelfuls of dirt. I wish I could imagine him reborn in flowers and plants sprung from his body. I wish I could promise myself that I would plant something on his grave, but I knew that I might only do it once and find reasons to forget it. I'd like my ashes to be buried in one of those green cemeteries next to a brook. No funeral.

As for funerals in general, I've sometimes had a little frisson of pleasure at the thought that it isn't me. Isn't me who choked in the night on a cough drop and had a heart attack. It isn't me who bent over to lace his sneaker for a run and fell face down on the pavement. But now it was different. I had seen Lucian with his urine bag and his wool cap, his face covered with stubble, and I was horrified. And what horrified me was that I was slowly moving towards that state. I didn't feel a saving distance between us. But Hannah was right, I had to go.

To encourage myself in the proper thoughts, I took out the packet of Christmas letters Lucian had sent me over the years. Nothing Christmassy—or Jewish for that matter—just lively descriptions of life with Gabriella. One I particularly liked had a picture of a family of ducklings on their lawn by the lake. Apparently the duck had laid her eggs in the bushes and when they hatched she wasn't able to get them down the very steep incline to the water. There must have been a drop-off too. Eventually Lucian carried them down, the mother duck following along anxiously. He was a good man, Lucian. He cared about people. I want to stir up my feeling for him but I can't find it. Only a slight trace of anger at him for removing himself. With him and George gone, there'll be just Gabriella and the memories of her much-loved brother, Primo.

At the cemetery I think I somehow expected a crowd like the one that followed his coffin. Would a reader nowadays understand the reference? You'd think as an Italian he would at least know the name and be able to say by rote: a great writer Primo Levi, one of the greatest in our time. But what would it mean to him? What remnants of a moral vision are left in our modern consumerist Italy? The economic miracle without a soul.

By now only the grandchildren of survivors are alive and the very old like me. Of course I had read Primo's books about Auschwitz. I'd admired his lucidity, his absence of rage at his persecutors, wondered how he could sustain these things; apparently he couldn't. In the end he succumbed, hurled himself down the stairwell of his mother's house. People said it was a delayed reaction to Auschwitz. That made it murder, not suicide, and allowed him to remain a hero. One can think that one is suffering at facing the future and instead be suffering because of one's past. I think he said that, though he didn't mean it in the Freudian sense. Then too he thought a lot about suicide. He talks in particular about an Austrian philosopher tortured by the Gestapo. This man, Amery, unable to forget what he'd been through, became incapable of finding joy in life, in living itself. That makes me feel that I am on the right track in soaking myself in whatever pleasure I find.

Just now a great flock of starlings went by, turning the sky dark with the beating of wings. Off to a new roosting place, I suppose. Primo found solace reciting Dante's Ulysses canto in which, if I remember correctly, Ulysses wants to sail to the ends of the known earth. Was hubris his sin?

It was enough to see the rabbi recite the *kaddish* to throw me back to that awful day. Back then, another spring morning, Hannah couldn't stop crying. Primo had called her in despair a few days before his death, and she had responded to him as if he had a headache, lecturing him on setting an example for the rest of them, the survivors.

"You couldn't have known," I told her. It seemed impossible that the man who had looked at the worst human beings can do to each other, that this man had done violence to himself. SAVED BUT DROWNED the newspapers trumpeted. TURIN MOURNS THE MAESTRO. But his funeral itself was like a silent movie. There were no noisy speeches. The widow in black and dark glasses walked behind him. So did she, of course, Gabriella. Delayed homicide, the rabbi had called it, so that he could be buried with honor. The Jews, like the Christians and Muslims, think of suicide as a sin and bury suicides in a separate unconsecrated part of the cemetery.

Hannah thought it wasn't the camps that had destroyed him; she insisted it was a love problem, an affair with a German woman. This seemed strange but she insisted, though she wouldn't tell me how she knew. And just now there was a biography that hinted at the same thing. His sister hated it, of course, and I put both biographies away somewhere and now I can't find them. I have some bookshelves set under the gable windows. I put them there when I was agile enough to crawl in and retrieve them. Anyway, I thought that Primo was worn down by the difficulties of living virtually imprisoned by his aged blind mother. Living with her was as much a litmus test of character as living in the Lager. Later, one of his biographers said, there had been a woman. I think he said a German woman, though I can't remember if he thought it was a love affair. Primo tended to have Platonic relations.

Now grave keepers have taken the fake grass from the grave and Lucian's coffin is lowered down. The rabbi chants the twenty-third psalm. I had wondered if there would be a nod to his Jewish roots. Then there were three short speeches at the grave side, one about his work for the World Health Organization, making films showing the correct way to plant and harvest crops in developing countries; another about his past as a Red on the Hollywood blacklist; and a third by a close friend who told about the wonderful rose garden Lucian had created near his country house on the lake outside Rome— almost a hundred species.

The roses lifted my spirits slightly but I kept looking down at the simple black coffin and remembering Edger Allan Poe's fear of being buried alive. If I had spoken I'd have told about Lucian's love of conversation. His memory was still intact, probably the only thing that was, and he loved to reminisce about his time in Hollywood and Mexico. You probably think the worse of me for not speaking, but since my mother died, I've hated funerals and avoided them whenever I could.

I think strain makes my memory worse. I mean stress, the stress of Lucian's funeral. Gabriella with pain with her leg, used an elegant cane. I need a brain cane. And while I'm thinking of it, it is really silly to keep calling her by an assumed name. Anyone who knows anything about Primo Levi will know she is his sister. And I have only good things to say about her. She is still beautiful, fine featured, elegant.

When Hannah and I came to visit she would always be wearing something Matisse-like, decorative. We always brought a catalogue from a recent exhibit—she particularly enjoyed the one on ephemera; which I think was at the Museo de Roma. She liked the idea that artists spent weeks constructing these floats or castles only to blow them up in a day's festivities. But mostly I think she liked it that for a little while, Lucian's flood of reminiscences would stop and she could hear about something that interested her.

As he got older and sicker, he seemed more desperate to pass on his memories. He showed us the whitewashed pueblo with red flowers in front where he lived with his common-law wife and her children. His other family, as he called it. The Mexican woman, short with a wide open face and her children holding on to her apron. Gabriella didn't seem to mind. And then they would joke about their two analysts, telling them they were suited to each other.

"The best boyfriend she's had yet," Lucian said and they laughed and we all felt young for a moment.

Did I tell you that already? Yes, I think so. And then he'd tell us how when he came back to California he had to produce movies under an assumed name. A friend of his, a woman, had written a very good book, *Reds on the Blacklist* or was it *The Red and the Blacklist*? It can't matter much. All about how difficult it was to get reestablished when the witch hunt had died down.

He told us a lot of other things too. A lot about his best friend George Oppen, who had been in Mexico with him and had introduced him to Gabriella—but I don't remember much of that. I'm not even sure about his introducing Lucian to Gabriella. I'd met George when I was visiting some film friends in California. George was still a believer in Comrade Mao, and that fascinated me. He was also a friend of that lunatic anti-Semite Ezra Pound.

I had the feeling during those years that I should have had a communist period as repentance for being born privileged and wealthy. George was born privileged too, of course. His family owned half the big movie palaces in San Francisco. After he was expelled from college for staying out all night with his girlfriend, (later his wife), Mary, his parents tried to keep them close by giving him a movie palace and by dressing Mary and covering her with jewels. I sometimes think of George and Mary as another version—a version in a different universe—of me and Hannah, one rich and one poor. But of course, being from a dirt poor Jewish family in Romania and being from a Midwestern farm aren't at all the same, especially when one of them, having dropped out of school, got an education riding around France in a horse-drawn wagon supported by a trust fund and the other got her education in Auschwitz!

But honestly, what most interested me about George was the fact that six members of his immediate family had committed suicide—his mother, his sister, his aunt. I don't remember the others. He wrote me once that Mary saved him from his Byzantine family. I thought of doing a film about him but kept putting it off, doing my social comedies instead. It probably wouldn't have done well here—a Jewish American poet who celebrates everyday things. *Materials* was the name of the book that won the Pulitzer Prize. He wrote most of it in Mexico before he came back. He'd had a dream about things rusting and realized it was his mind that was rusting. He had a way of moving between his mind and things, reconsidering and changing his impressions. It's awful for anyone to have the memory battery run down, but especially for him, left only with the things themselves.

I compare myself to him, both of us getting lost on streets we know, forgetting the face of someone we know. No, it's too depressing.

Let's see, what have I forgotten lately?

Yesterday I forgot to tell Hannah her niece Sarah called while she was out. She was just going to be out a few minutes and I was sure I'd remember it. What else? Well, I forgot my doctor's appointment. I also forgot that I was supposed to get my hair cut. Hannah did it for me. No need to go out, really. And I like her fussing over me. Just now she came into my study and casually riffled through my last few pages. Not something she usually does.

"I hope you're not thinking of publishing this," she said.

"No, I'm just thinking of getting things down, unloading my brain before it signs off."

"But when you write those things about Lucian, can you imagine Gabriella reading about your seeing his urine bag?"

"She can barely read the headlines with a magnifier."

"That's an exaggeration. And these days things can get on a blog or a tweet and go all around the globe in a second. Someone might call her up."

"Stop already. It's very unlikely that anyone will read this. I'm not Proust."

She laughs. "She might think I was egging you on because of that quarrel I had with Lucian."

"That was twenty years ago. You should have made it up long ago. You both cared for each other and he loved you. He was upset about your talking to, who was it?"

"His niece."

"That got him into trouble with his family." Honestly I couldn't remember what had been so important. But I knew that Hannah couldn't keep a secret. All secrets were on the same plane with her. They had to be poured into someone's ear like the poison in *Hamlet*. Maybe the habit of witnessing simply took over. I would have liked to see her run for mayor of Rome, running against corruption. Her friend Rina was a Roman senator. I remember one day I had lunch with Rina—a beautiful woman, by the way—and she introduced me to another senator, saying here is the only one who knows the difference between *cultura* and *spazzatura*. Culture and Garbage! She was some woman, that Rina! Her husband was a big publisher—I think Mondadori.

I was curious about why she lived separately. She cupped her breasts and laughed. "He wants my milk. I need my milk for myself."

Her voice was like a lioness purring. Another day, I accompanied her to the palace. She'd been invited to dinner with the president and was bringing him her book. Like a real tourist, I took her picture with one of those handsome guards. Maybe I'm the only person who knows those things. Plump little moments to swell out a future biography. A researcher will be happy to find them. She did win the *Strega*, after all, and her memoir of the war years is brilliant.

Hannah is tapping her foot impatiently. "We weren't talking about my quarrel with Lucian. We were talking about your airing your negative thoughts. And in any case, I couldn't make up with Lucian because he and she joked to people about you and Claudia—*La Dentista*, Gabriella called her, and people would laugh. Listen, *Caro*, I don't want to go on with this. Erminia is coming soon and I have to go to the market."

"*Vai con calma. Non ti preoccipi.*"

After she goes, I think about what she said. I suppose I should suppress some of this. But not now. Some of what I am saying is libelous, no doubt. If I remember correctly libel is anything that gives a negative picture. Truth is no defense. I like the sound of that and roll it on my tongue. Truth is no defense.

Yesterday or maybe just some hours ago—time has gotten a funny way of compressing itself—I found an old shoe box in the storage space next to the couch in the entry to our apartment. Erminia uses the space to store the ironing board and we used to put our suitcases there between trips. I don't suppose we'll be going anywhere soon. But in all the jumble of things I found a box of my mother's old letters from friends. I leafed through and read a couple.

They seemed to be from younger friends, mostly artists or writers she had invited to dinner, who had told her their problems. Reading them, I feel as if she were still alive. Her friends obviously don't realize how troubled she is. They ask her what to do about getting a gallery, finding a publisher, dealing with a difficult child. I have a vague memory of people at her funeral talking about how wise she was, implying that we, the children—the comments were mostly addressed to my older brother—must be suffering from having lost such a mother.

The thing is, children miss their mothers terribly even if they are monsters, even if they beat them black and blue, tie them to the bedpost, starve them. Even if the children could run away, they don't. My mother wasn't like that, of course. If anything she left me alone too much. I had the idea that she hired a nanny when I was born. It would have been an English Nanny because she wanted us to be bilingual. And after that, she paid us no attention. But now I think that is wrong. It's nice to know your memory can deceive you.

Did you know, by the way, that Maurice Sendak, the great writer of children's books, said he never wanted to have children because it was too much trouble? That's how I thought my mother felt. But yesterday—since I saw the sunrise in my window mirror, I know it's a new day—I found a little leather notebook with "Baby's Sayings and Doings" engraved on it in gold. And there it was with my name inside and the date of my birth, 1922, and my weight, five pounds. I hadn't known that I was so small. It must have worried mother because she notes my weight week after week. She had a delicate script and used brown ink. She wrote in straight lines, ignoring the broader spaces provided by the notebook. It could almost be a work of art. Her words sculpt my living body. By nine weeks I weigh nine pounds. By three months I am twelve pounds. The jottings continue until I am five, long past the time when she might have been anxious about my weight, You see, don't you, that this means she cared about me. Ruling off the tiny pages and writing in her careful artist's script.

Did I tell you she was a painter? Never a very successful one, but a painter nonetheless. And now I have established that she cared. A little further on, she records my feeding schedule, seven feedings a day. She didn't nurse me—I know that. She told me she couldn't because my father thought nursing caused breast cancer.

I was standing up in my playpen at twelve months, waving goodbye, saying Mama, Nana, Dada. By then I was eating a variety of things, including custard and mashed vegetables. Wouldn't you say that shows…? Or maybe if you were unbiased it wouldn't show anything. By fourteen months I'm walking and listening to music. I like *Au claire de la Lune* and Italian and American nursery songs. When my nurse sings them, I bounce up and down rhythmically. Ah, so already I am a little artist, or perhaps a musician. My mother notes that her friend Margaret came over one day and played on the piano—it must have been the grand piano at Todi. She told my mother that I listened and tried to sing. Also for the first time I played with a little boy, Pietro.

And at around fifteen months I submitted to toilet training. That would be young, I think, by today's standards and of course I don't remember it. Then comes something I do remember: my first accident. I fell into a cactus plant and she had to pick out the spines one by one. When I think of it I see an enormous jade-green cactus, or maybe a garden of them, and me dressed only in my diaper, coming nearer and nearer. Mother used to remind me how long it took to pluck out the spines with a tweezer and how miserable I was.

But most of her observations in the baby book were positive or neutral. I liked to look people over before making friends, and so mother directs visitors to play with my panda or a toy until I come over. That usually happens sooner rather than later, for I am very *inquisitive.* That is underlined in red. And then there is a tiny portrait of a baby's head surrounded by a wreath of flowers. Could you guess that such a mother would later kill herself? Doesn't she sound both caring and sane, or have I missed something? I read a little more. The pediatrician pronounces me anemic, prescribes iron, beef juice, liver. My mother is upset to think that this could happen; she had felt sure, she says, that I was getting every care and was "perfectly normal." Well, maybe she's a little controlling, anxious, but still, I am fascinated by her looking at me, watching me. She faithfully records my first cold, my response to commands, my trying and not succeeding to eat with a spoon, how she lets me push the food around. I like this young mother. She notices everything. True, she is on the alert for signs of talent. But so are a lot of mothers. She is enchanted by my reactions to sophisticated music. I love jazz and Mozart or Schoenberg. I now like to look at picture books. Mother records my increasing vocabulary, also my sunbaths with an ultraviolet lamp. Oh, that's not a good one; I guess I'm a candidate for melanoma.

By sixteen months I look at myself in the mirror, then look at my mother, bemused. Already a young Derrida, or was it Lacan with all the mirror business? There is one note that makes me slightly uncomfortable. She says I follow her from room to room. Where was my nanny? Maybe on her day off. I sense there is something else going on. But what? The surprise of finding this little diary is wearing off. I am almost finished. Tired.

Then on the next page I see that she takes a two-week vacation and says I am almost hysterical when she gets back. After that, Mother says she is feeding me herself and she continues to let me play with the food, something my new German Nanny, no doubt obsessed with cleanliness, didn't permit. Even if Mother does this to compensate for finding me undone by her absence, her doing it is the important thing. So it isn't true, the story I told myself for years, that she saw me only before I went to sleep. She couldn't have observed all these things if she'd just looked in on me once a day. No, she seems to have been truly engrossed in my progress.

But still something seems to me to be glossed over. When she mentions that I am less hysterical when the second nanny is fired than when the first was, suddenly I remember. The first one was fired after she let me fall on my head, going headfirst down a slide. Mother used to tell me about it. It must have been traumatic. I know she told me that I had to stay in bed so long that I forgot how to walk. Could she have been censoring her journal? I don't want to think that. And she does note my hysteria after she goes away for a two week vacation. Did I say that already? I'd love to know what she means by "hysterical" exactly. She only notes that I forgot my toilet training and was off my feed. Whatever my infant state, it seemed to her that I made less fuss the second time she changed my caretaker. A Freudian might say this set up life-long problems with separation, perhaps later making Hannah suffer what I'd suffered. That's the kind of thing they like to speculate about. But I'm tired now. I go out on the terrace to lie down in the sun.

Things are bursting into bloom here and buds are everywhere. Even my recalcitrant olive is flourishing. I think about going for a walk but Hannah would be angry that I went without her. I wish she didn't worry so much. The back streets of Rome are like a village, particularly in this neighborhood. But they are not. Maybe they just seem that way. I imagine going to the fruit and vegetable store. I can almost see it from our front door. I don't think I'd get lost. I'd go in and feel the melons, go next door and buy some *prosciutto*. But no, she'd be angry. Instead I start thinking about Primo in Auschwitz. It comes into my mind without being asked. At the same time I see a seagull catch an air current and soar by me, coming down on the chimney and looking around with its red eye. Strange things bubble up in my memory, like the old men Primo describes, going to the toilet and having no paper to wipe themselves. How they suffered from the humiliation. Old men like me now.

It was all about dirt. The old men were "dirty Jews." Their shit ran down their scrawny legs like brown water. Everything was made as humiliating as possible, the dirty rags they—I almost said we—were forced to wear, the clogs with broken soles, the shaving of hair to destroy the lice. All to humiliate them, disgusting Jews in their second childhood, weak as babies, dropping dead from exhaustion during roll call. Hannah suffered those things too. My Hannah, and she was just a child, but she never wanted to kill herself, though of course the thought of it must have crossed her mind.

One of her friends there ran into the electric fence. Another tried to escape and was hung in front of all of them. Actually, she—I think her name was Ella—defied the hangman by putting her own head in the noose and stepping off the platform. Robbing them of a victory. How different from the poet who put her head in an oven after turning on the gas, with her children in the next room—or my mother in her bed. I want so much to understand, but the suicides still make me sick. Worse than sick; furious, in a rage. Anne Sexton, for instance. Didn't she go out to the car in which she planned to gas herself with nothing on but a luxurious fur coat? Such a coat might have saved a prisoner's life. Her daughter had to cope with that display every day of her life. I can't manage, I can't do it, can't forgive.

The sun rose so gradually this morning I was almost afraid it wasn't going to come up. It was dark when I got up, with the moon hanging in a corner of the sky, still quite bright. *La lune ne garde aucune rancune.*

One thing that is good about geriatric sex is its delicious slowness. It would be good to die that way, like going to sleep after. But I'm afraid I won't be so lucky. That's why people make suicide pacts, I suppose, to be sure—like coming together. It's not the dying that frightens me so much. It's the thought of... of what? In the night I saw shadows in our room and heard something gnawing and skittering inside the wall. It frightened me to the point of wanting to scream. Instead I called Hannah. I felt as though some Eldritch horror was positively coming to get me.

Just before morning is the worst time for my hallucinations—as Hannah calls them. Her doctor told her they're common in cases of dementia. Sometimes I see a shadowy figure approaching the bed. I try to remember that it's probably Hannah getting up to go to the bathroom, but I can't shake off the fear that it's a murderer. If you want to know how it feels, think of Tony Perkins in *Psycho*, approaching the shower. Or the Mother with the knife. How strange for that to come to mind. Little bits of it surface slowly. At first I only remembered that Tony was living with his old mother. Then I recalled with a sick feeling in my stomach, that he had become his mother, that she inhabited half of his mind! My romantic vision of a suicide pact turned into murder. Tony, insanely jealous of his mother's lover, had poisoned them both. No, that was not at all the double suicide I was thinking about but still, two dead—mother and lover.

Am I jealous of the lovers Hannah might have after I die? Yes, I'm afraid I am. I hate to think of her bringing them here where we started out as young lovers. Maybe I should talk to her about it. Tell her that of course I'll leave her the apartment with the stipulation that she won't bring any future husband or lovers here. Would she honor that? I doubt it. And who am I to ask her anything like that after my years with Claudia?

I wish I had a piercing searchlight that could see into her brain, the way those new machines do, and spy on her thoughts. I could pronounce the names of her boyfriends— she'd had plenty when I was with Claudia—girlfriends too for that matter, and see what parts lit up. But now? The one time I mentioned my painful thoughts, she laughed, reminding me that she'd had one heart attack and might very well have another. Didn't I ask her to take me back so I could care for her?

Elders is what they call us now, *anziani.* As in "respect your elders." It seems instead of respect we are now the chosen targets for all sorts of crimes. Hannah came back from lunch with her friend Arianne with a particularly egregious example.

Arianne's grandson had called her on the phone late at night and saluted her with "grandma," a word that makes her quiver with pleasure. She worships all her grandchildren. But she couldn't quite tell if it was Guido or Jacobo. When she asked if this was Guido, the boy said yes. Guido's's voice had been changing for several months so she attributed his slight hoarseness to that or possibly a cold.

They chatted for a few minutes. Arianne thought he might be fishing for a birthday present although she had already given him an anticipatory one, a guitar. Quite expensive too. They chatted for a few minutes—Oh, I already said that and it probably didn't matter that they chatted, except that when she asked about it, he was comfortable talking about the guitar and how he was enjoying the touring band.

Then out of the blue in a tiny voice he told her he'd had an accident. He'd been coming home from a party on the outskirts of Rome with some friends, and the driver had had too much to drink, so he took over. He had himself had two beers but he assured her he felt perfectly alert and what happened wasn't his fault. The car in front of them stopped short and he rear-ended it. Then the police arrived and gave him a breath test. He failed it by a fraction, but when they took him to the station and let him take it again, he passed.

"What? You're at the police station?" Arianne was aghast. "Did you call your parents?"

"They told me that I have only one call. So I thought..."

"Of course," Arianne said, secretly thrilled that the boy would trust her to help him. "But I don't understand; why aren't they letting you go?"

"It's complicated, Grandma, the people in the Audi were foreigners. Their insurance will cover the damages, but the Hertz company insists on being paid back before they leave the country. The judge said he won't release me until they receive the money, and if I don't get it, they'll have to keep me overnight with the common prisoners."

Arianne felt she was out of her depth, so she called her husband who asked to speak to someone at the station. Michelle, a well-spoken man who said he was the public defender got on the phone and patiently confirmed what the boy had said. The public defender said he was making every effort to keep the accident and the "impaired judgment" off Guido's record. He thought that the experience had already "taught him a lesson." He concluded by asking who would be taking care of this; the money, $2,400, was needed immediately. Could they manage?

"Of course," Arianne's husband said, and the public defender told them step-by-step how to wire money from a store *in centro*. In the center. He gave them the name, spelling it out carefully, "E as in Edgar, D as in Dan, G as in..." Then the last name and the number. "Be sure not to mention what it is for," the public defender said. "Don't mention the impairment, just say it is a loan to a friend." He ended by leaving the number where he could be reached and promised to call back promptly. He promised that Guido would be released that afternoon.

Oh no, this is no good. I can't expect you to get excited about people you don't know. And besides, it is all a lie. It wasn't Arianne who answered the phone, it was me, though Hannah had told me to let the answering machine pick up. I answered the phone because I was bored and couldn't think of anything to write in my journal. The "boy" that called was pretending to be Hannah's nephew, Guido. He was visiting from Florence or was it America? From the moment I heard his voice, I was confused. It didn't sound like anyone I knew. But I often forget what people sound like now, and I wanted to manage this conversation really well to show Hannah I was still capable. So I chatted enthusiastically about Guido's music with him. When he told me about his accident, rear ending some tourists from Lebanon, I was first in shock and then lost in the flurry of detail. The main thing I gathered was that it wasn't his fault, that he was in jail, and that he needed money quickly.

I panicked. What would Hannah do? For a moment it crossed my mind that he was too young to drive, but then I forgot it. If he was calling like this he must have gotten a license since we saw him last. To be honest, I hadn't paid much attention to him when he came over for tea one day with his mother to visit with Hannah. I tried to keep my attention focused on Guido's problem. It all hinged on money which is one of the things I find hardest now. Was it twenty-four euros he needed or twenty-four hundred? By now the man who called himself a public defender had gotten on the phone and gone over the whole story. It was the bigger sum—a mistake would have been unfortunate. The point seemed to be that Guido needed it right away or else his failure in some test, a breath test I think, would be on his record forever and ever. Where would I get the money? I was searching for my key with the idea of going to the bank with Hannah's bank card—she'd taken mine away—and explaining the whole thing and persuading them I needed to use her card, that it was an emergency. I was waiting for the elevator outside our front door when Hannah came back.

"'What are you doing?" she asked me, then she answered herself. "Were you coming to look for me again? I told you I'd be home in an hour and its only forty-five minutes. Come, let's go inside and have some tea."

I babbled out my story, tripping over my tongue, feeling completely mortified.

"Oh Bubbi, can't you see it's a scam? And what a cruel one." I hung my head. "Didn't you remember that he's only fifteen, that he has no license?"

"I almost did…but then…" I felt as if I were about to cry. Was this the same man who had directed movies and given lectures to students?

"Never mind, then." Hannah said kindly. "It was such an inventive scam that I'm sure a lot of people would have been taken in."

"If I were still twenty I would have known. At eighty-eight the mind doesn't function in the same way." I waved away my age with an elegant flick of my wrist. I wished she'd stop looking at me so pityingly. We went inside and she made me a cup of chamomile tea.

"If I were still twenty," I repeated, "I would have been more alert. It was the word 'uncle' that did me in."

"Of course it would. Family—what is more important?" she paused and I saw the faraway look she has when she is thinking about her novels and trying out a scene or a bit of dialogue. And it *was* amazing how inventive this scam was. It was like something that might happen in a novel. Full of intense emotional drama.

A little later, I was reclining in my chair under a throw when Hannah handed me the paper. "Don't brood, Renzo. It's bad for digestion. Nothing happened after all; we're lucky. But in the future..." I could hear her pausing. She had wanted to urge me to remember something, but she wasn't sure I could. "I'll write down some questions you could ask. If anything like this happens again. Above all, don't lead with information. Let them tell you." She kissed my head and took the tea things into the kitchen.

I spread the paper on my lap and studied the photo of a big ship lying on its side. Actually it may have been a picture of something else, but I'm sure it was something that could start a novel. In the case of the ship, the press made it into a theatrical with the cowardly play boy resembling Berlusconi and the upright sailor like our head of state, Monti, who told the fleeing captain to get the hell back on the ship. We love struggles between good and evil. It must be something genetic, taken in somehow with mother's milk. Look at the Americans now, ankle deep in moral mud with their ridiculous candidates bellowing and roaring their love of Jesus while committing every possible sin. I love the recent story in which the newspapers excuse a former senator's affair because, after all, he asked his wife for permission to have an open marriage.

Wait a minute—didn't I once try to get Hannah to do that with me? Put her on a starvation dict with just enough to keep her alive. Is it possible the Muslims have the right idea? Every wife has to have equal time and attention. I'd like to interview some of those wives! Even young and strong I doubt I could have done it, and I don't mean just the sex.

Still, if it were customary to have several wives I could have moved Claudia right in without Hannah's being able to make much of a fuss. Once in Paris, I was attending a conference on film, memory, and history and went to a panel discussion of *Guests of the Sheik* by Elizabeth Furnea. At that time I was rather taken with doing a film about harem life. I loved the idea of all those women lounging by baths, like the odalisques in the paintings of Ingres, who was attracted to the sensuality of all that lovely flesh. Furnea found that, contrary to our Western prejudice, many of the women enjoyed their harem life, particularly the opportunity to gossip and go on outings together. Raising their children together apparently relieved much of the isolation of family life in the West. And of course the sheik took care of them when they were sick or grew old.

It didn't seem half-bad and was certainly a great source of male fantasy. Imagine choosing a different woman every night. And each of them showing only me—the sheik—their fancy clothes, silk teddies, lacy bras, and gold jewelry hidden under their black *abayas*. Naturally I didn't mention my fantasies to the gaggle of feminist scholars who were inveighing against genital mutilation, which of course I opposed as well.

After the panel I ended up at dinner with four young men from Mali, a country somewhat to the north of Nigeria—who had actually seen harem life close up. They were the most amazing looking people, black as ebony with gleaming white teeth. The oldest was writing about his family's experience with polygamy. His grandfather, he told me, had 58 wives and 256 grandchildren, his father only four. It was terribly difficult for him to be allowed only one. He felt diminished, limited by European law.

I asked him how the wives got along. His mother was the youngest, and the elder wives were quite jealous and would play tricks, trying to get her in trouble, but his father was very much in love with her and would always laugh and pull her onto his lap and kiss her. Sometimes if one of the elder wives was particularly angry, he would look serious and promise that he'd punish her later. But he never did.

If I'd been a woman I would have been fascinated by the young men, their skin that invited touching, like a fine fabric. But not dry, more like a dolphin's wet darkness. I could imagine them running down to the ocean naked.

How much bravery is needed to return to a sinking ship in the dark? Primo Levi says it is impossible to judge ahead of time what one is capable of doing in a crisis. I could almost swear that I wouldn't have gone back. I say almost because I agree for the moment that one can never be sure. I was a coward from childhood. Or at least that's how I see myself. I remember one incident at Mardi Gras in Venice, I was wearing a Little Lord Fauntleroy outfit, my golden ringlets down to my shoulders. The suit was brown velvet with a antique lace collar. My mother thought I was adorable but it served only as a red flag to the local bulls.

I was set upon and hit, not very hard, by three slightly larger boys. They had socks filled with rice. I was petrified and ran back to our hotel in tears. Much later I'd find my sanctuary in language, knowing things, speaking and understanding many languages. Apparently in the Lager, the Italian prisoners died soon after they arrived, partly because they couldn't understand German and couldn't find out the things they needed to know—not facts in the lives of Proust or Tolstoy, but the things that would keep them alive: how to get shoes and illegal food, how to deal with illness.

Hannah, though she only spoke Romanian and Yiddish, was good at survival, having to practice these tactics in her village. And she had her older sister, Leah, with her, a woman of strong character who maintained her humanity and tried always to shield her, even volunteering to be selected in her place. I couldn't imagine doing that, though I'd like to believe if Hannah were sick or threatened, I'd put my body between her and a bullet.

Somehow even with all my freight of eighty-eight years, I wasn't able to grow my humanity to its fullest. Early on I developed a protective shell. I didn't suffer the horrors of the camps, but certainly my life was full of suffering. I feel embarrassed at still pointing my finger at my mother, making it her fault. Someone once said that a suicide leaves its skeleton in the survivors' closet. Was I fated to seek out a person who was as damaged as I felt myself, despite all my languages and honors? Primo insists that suffering doesn't make the prisoners saints as some have called them.

Critics, when Hannah presents them with a new work, treat it like Holy Scripture—particularly the one in which she tells her mother about her life, knowing her mother will disapprove—but if I were to describe the way my mother ravaged my psyche, I'd be criticized for whining, for cowardice. There seems to be no way out for me.

Primo Levi himself insists that the camp inmates became more and more like their tormenters the longer they stayed. Isn't that true in the outside world too? A beaten child beats his wife or children, a drunk spawns an enabler, someone who simpers and colludes with his oppressor. But Primo also says that you can't judge unless you have been there. To say we are all murderers deep inside—a trope picked up by some artists— is false, a moral disease that serves only to muddy the truth.

When I met Hannah I felt as if I shared her suffering, taking it on, jettisoning my own past, but I couldn't keep it up, could I? An uglier motive for my care taking was my envy. I wanted to gain merit as a saint, if not in the camps, here at home.

Was it Virginia Woolf who said that when you have a toothache the whole world contracts to that point of pain in your mouth? Something like that anyway. And when the on-going blitz set off firecrackers in her brain, she stuffed her pockets full of stones. I picture them as those black smooth ones so friendly to the touch, maybe warmed by the sun along the banks of the river. Was she tempted by the comforting roundness to stay awhile? By that point, she was too afraid of her madness, the voices in her head.

I see suicides are piling up in my remembrances. Arshile Gorky, Anne Sexton, Gina's daughter, Virginia Woolf, Primo Levi, and like a Greek chorus after each one, my mother, my mother, my mother. I think I said that if you want to escape being dragged down by the stones of death, you have to find pleasure. The thing is, for the most part their pleasure receptors were high. They didn't sit around burdened by gloom. Gorky for instance could be transported by the thought of his mother's apron. My mother was thrown into raptures by the purple radiance of a desert sunset, or even the saturated color of a single flower. I remember as a child asking her to show me what she saw, thinking that I was defective, that I was missing some sense. And it didn't stop at colors. She also smelled and tasted things more intensely than I did.

It occurs to me that autistic children are exquisitely aware of certain things. That's why they fiddle with their fingers or bang their heads, which may hurt but it's regular and, more important, they can regulate it themselves. Filmmaking was a little like that for me. I could doctor the images the way people do now in Photoshop, adding more yellow, more blues and purples, cutting and cropping, flattering myself that I was seeing more than the ordinary person, inside and out. I specialized in flashbacks. The memories of the characters became mine to manipulate.

Well, I had my painful tooth extracted, one of my yesterdays. The doctor saved the tooth to show me. There was a hole in the root below the gum line, and the whole inside was eaten out, so brittle there was no way to fill it. It was hollow like the hollow men in Tom Eliot's great poem, except that there was no straw around to fill it. An anti-Semite, old Tom, and he behaved badly to his wife as well, if you like odd facts. The hollow men make me think of the scarecrow in *The Wizard of Oz*, setting out so bravely to get his head filled with brains, and of Jack Pumpkinhead, getting a fresh head when the old one wore out.

I was reading again to my little neighbor Roberto and we talked for a while about there being no death in Oz, though you could be cut into pieces and hidden. Dorothy should always wear the magic belt, he said. Then she'd be safe. I asked him if he'd like to make a magic belt for himself. He said yes, and I told him I had the perfect thing for it. I had a beautiful piece of gold cloth—in fact it was a shower curtain that Hannah hated and that we were going to replace. We took it out on the terrace in the sun, along with a gardener's sheers and some fabric swatches that we could cut up to make diamonds and some superglue to attach them. He couldn't quite manage the sheers but he did very well with the glue and we decided that some of the diamonds should be changed to emeralds or sapphires, so he got to color them with indelible magic markers, being very careful not to get any color on his shirt. When we finished I made a clasp out of safety pins and put it on him. He took a deep breath and I felt the tension going out of his body, then he leaned against me and very lightly kissed my shoulder.

It occurs to me that I haven't said much about sex. I haven't admitted for instance that I think of it constantly, am always touching myself though I'm afraid to work at it very hard for fear of a heart attack. I get scared when I feel a throbbing in my temples, as though I am going to rupture something. Some people would certainly say that sex oughtn't to be a concern for a person of my age.

"Eighty-eight! My god," they say, "you should be glad that you're still alive."

They wouldn't care if I had my balls cut right off. I find myself touching them at times during the day just to reassure myself that they're still there. My mother was only in her forties when she died, but she was bedridden off and on before that with some kind of a fatigue syndrome; it never was clear whether it was psychological. But it made her think a lot about what she was missing. Drawing was the one thing that seemed to ease her pain. She could draw propped up on her pillows, leaning her pad on her breakfast tray. She had one with folding legs that kept it from pressing on her.

Much later, I found some of the drawings: big penises spouting spunk. I was shocked. No one, of whatever their age, likes to think of his mother having sex. I wasn't as prudish as one of my friends who found his mother in bed with a man at the nursing home, but still. The most disturbing of her drawings was one of Christ on the cross with a big erection. Was the absence of sex crucifying him? Remember that D. H. Lawrence novella with Jesus and some pagan priestess? Or was that the Spanish writer? The one who wrote *The Stone Raft*? I've forgotten his name.

My mother had scrawled some words in the margins: "I want someone, male or female, to come and make love to me."

There were other things as well. They made me wonder if Hannah really still wanted it too, aside from hugging me in bed and letting me put my head on her breasts—still nice by the way—white and welcoming with large pink nipples made for suckling. But lately she hasn't signaled that she wants to go further. That might be my fault, however. I haven't wanted to confront my diminishing powers, or frighten myself with the pounding in my head.

It is the waiting that is unbearable, someone wrote recently. This suspension of time, waiting for something to happen and knowing you are unable to struggle against it.

I am getting too broody. I'll get Hannah to take me to a big show of Tizianos, mostly from the Prado. I haven't fully dressed myself for days, just lounging about in my robe and pj's, but the idea of seeing the Tizianos rouses me and, looking in the mirror after I dress, I rather like the distinguished older man who stares back at me. I slept well last night and the pouches under my eyes are diminished. If I put on a little bit of Hannah's makeup, they won't be visible at all—or hardly.

"Don't rush down the steps," Hannah cautions me. "Remember what happened to Lucian on his last visit."

I did remember: he almost fell and we had to help him up. "It's the last time I'm going to risk my neck on these damn stairs," he muttered under his breath, reverting to the scrappy

Brooklyn boy he had been when I met him. "But your terrace is so glorious with everything in bloom."

I don't know if I've said that Lucian was a devoted gardener. Maybe that is connected to his having spent years showing peasant farmers in third world countries how to urge something green from parched earth. Then again, maybe there is no connection. When I used to go with him to his country villa in a little village on a lake near Rome, we would always stop at his favorite horticulturist and pick up pots of something special for his garden. I would help him carry them. It was always a treat to visit. He would throw open the windows one after another and the dazzling blue of the sunlit lake would suffuse the rooms with color. It was the stairs that did him in. The three-story house was built into a hill. He should have had his knees replaced, but he was a stubborn man, Lucian. I am lucky; I still can walk the full flight from the fifth floor up to the sixth. Our *attico* must be an add on, so the elevator doesn't go all the way up.

With my folding stool—Hannah carried it for me though I could do it perfectly well myself—I sat and drank in, devoured really, all that beautiful creamy flesh in the Tizianos. My favorite is the *Danaë*, with her lying back on her pillows, swooning, one hand limp between her legs while Jupiter rains down gold coins. His head, visible in the cloud, suggests that the painting is the dream of an old man. Danaë is ravished by his imagination. When we got home, I took Hannah to bed, still thinking of Danaë. Do you know that Stendhal recorded all the times he had sex and the number of his orgasms? Well, one for me then. Slower, less impetuous, but golden all the way through.

Another visit to the neurologist. Things seem to be more or less the same. I couldn't remember the name and address she gave me and had trouble spelling backwards—both things I had trouble with last time. I'm on a plateau, she says. No telling how long it will last. Hannah told her about my falling for the scam and she added a caveat: maybe my judgment is slightly impaired. But I think a lot of people could have fallen for it.

On the way back in the taxi Hannah kept looking at her watch. It turned out she was supposed to meet Carlo, a young director, about doing a film of her latest book. She had mentioned this before, but I have my doubts that it will happen since he sounds scattered and has been going to and fro—first trouble with money, then trouble with his wife.

"You're just jealous," Hannah said. "And I'm not going to humor you by telling you there is nothing in it. He's a handsome man, yes? I like him. You don't have a leg to stand on, you know, even if I were to fall in love with him, especially if I fell in love with him." Then she laughed in an unpleasant way. "But I'm not in love with him now, so you don't need to put on your doleful face. Stop!" she called out and the taxi driver screeched to a halt just beyond our corner. They always seem to overshoot.

I got out. I would have liked to be the one to pay the driver but lately Hannah has been doing all the money things, just because I made a mistake and gave a waiter fifty euros for a tip, by mistake instead of five. I felt humiliated as she got out and walked around to his front window and paid, then took my arm and walked me to the door. I stepped ahead and fumbled with my keys, suddenly not sure which was to the downstairs door.

"The big one," Hannah said impatiently. "You see how much bigger that one is." And she reached out, took the key, and opened the door.

Upstairs I didn't even want to try to disarm the alarm. I couldn't remember the code. I had trouble with that even before I started having memory problems. I never was at home with numbers. I had set it with a historical date, thinking I'd be sure to remember that. Was it 1492, the date Columbus set sail, or...? But before I could try it, Hannah brushed by me and punched in the numbers.

"I knew that," I said.

If you made a mistake—and I had made several—the alarm set off the most horrible wail. Our neighbors would open their doors and peek out, afraid that someone had broken in. It happens every few years that someone comes down from the roof and breaks one of the terrace doors. Or picks the lock which isn't very strong. I had gotten in the habit of hiding my valuables. I got so good at it, and we had so many nooks and crevices, that Hannah used to say if something happened to me, she'd never find them.

"You're tired," she said now as she opened the shutters and the sliding door and brought the back pillow for my terrace chair. She wanted me to amuse myself watching the gulls while she was out drowning in the midnight blue eyes of this punk producer.

I don't think of myself as a jealous man, except maybe of my brother. But this Don Carlo strikes me as a con artist or maybe just an enthusiast. He bought her book, loved it, and now this business about a film, *Moon Dreams* he wants to call it. I try to question her but she shrugs me off.

"You just like control," she says, "but this has nothing to do with you now."

I can't help reminding her of the films I made with her about her village, how I helped her, how without me she wouldn't be where she was now.

"I don't want to hear that ," she said. "Then was then, now is now. But if it will make you feel any better, I think he's gay."

She has a lot of gay friends, though being gay didn't stop one of them from sleeping with her when I was off with Claudia. I began to feel that she was taunting me, turning the tables now that I was weak. Standing there, I was about to cry from frustration when she turned affectionate, put her arms around me, and hugged me.

"It's you I love," she said, fluffing my chair pillow and pushing me down. "I can't help it. You are an irresistible man, you know that? Of course you do." She opened the big umbrella over the deck and stuck in the pin. "You were so sure of me you thought you could get me to accept that ridiculous Claudia as your second wife, the sort of woman we always made fun of, with only big tits on her résumé. Don Carlo at least has brains."

When she goes, I sit in my canvas chair and brood. Maybe the worst thing is that this Don Carlo is also in the movie business. It isn't exactly true that I'm not jealous. Certainly I was jealous as a child of my father—following the old Freudian script. I did everything I could to satisfy her and make her happy but it clearly wasn't enough. I could clean my room until it sparkled and pick up my wash, even though I knew the servants were supposed to do those things and could do them better. But she did let me brush her hair, and I was the only one who had that privilege.

Her hair was honey colored and thick like amber-colored silk spread over her shoulders. Afterwards she let me smooth a cream onto her shoulders and neck to keep them fresh and sometimes if she felt lonely she would invite me to lie with her in bed. That was what I imagined heaven to be—lying forever next to my mother, my face buried in her hair. Sometimes I got an erection and she would pretend to be shocked and banish me and "that nasty thing," at other times she would let me lie behind her and would move her back and buttocks against me while pretending to sleep.

In *liceo* I always had crushes on beautiful aloof girls and set myself to wooing them, but I don't think I was jealous until now. I hate it that Hannah isn't content with me and my aging body. To torment myself I make a list of things she complains about. I leave my shoes in the doorway and she trips over them in the night. I don't turn the knob fully and the door clicks open in the night if there is a wind. I leave the cabinets open. I was distracted and let a pot burn smoky black. When I make myself an egg—something she used to do for me—I don't rinse the pan out and egg sticks to it like glue. I won't get new heels on my shoes; I complain that they don't fit. I fart in bed a bugle call to the apocalypse. The list keeps growing; I cry thinking of it. All these little things add up. I'm sorry, I say, so sorry. I know how hard it must be for you.

Some hopeful news about Alzheimer's in the paper today. I was at Alfredo's lingering over my cappuccino and *cornetto* while Hannah went to Campo di Fiori to search for a melon she wanted to have for lunch with prosciutto. The melons in our local vegetable store weren't fully ripe, and we were having company: Arianne and her husband. We have been seeing relatively few people.

I used to do most of the fancy cooking. I made a fantastic spaghetti with clams, and my fried zucchini blossoms were famous. But recently I seemed to have lost my touch, cooking things too little or too much. It seemed easier to let Hannah do it—otherwise she just stood around carping. And she didn't laugh when I called her my *cuòco del dìetro*, roughly, "my back-side chef."

Anyway, apparently diseased brain cells can spread to their neighbors. I think they call it the Tao, or is that something in Buddhism? Maybe it's Tau—a protein of some sort. I just read about it a minute ago and already I've forgotten. But the point was that they can now concentrate on blocking the Tao/Tau, or whatever it is, and they might have a cure by 2025. Since it's too late for me in any case, I shut the paper and concentrate on the sensation of the cappuccino's warm foam against my lips. It gives me a pang to see the heart drawn in the foam. Alfredo's widow is keeping up his custom, but without the maestro of Via Giulia greeting us by belting out a passionate passage from *Tosca* or *Aida* while he sets down the tray, it's not the same. He has been the guardian, the soul of this great street for thirty years. He knew the history of all the important buildings and the families that lived in them.

A week before he died he sat at our table with us and proudly showed us an article about him and the existentialist poet Ingeborg Bachmann. She lived in the old Sacchetti Palace down by the river, and one night she went to sleep without putting out her cigarette. Alfredo went to deliver her espresso one morning and found her dead. At least that was the story. I mentally add her to my somewhat obsessive list of suicides, along with Tosca. I don't know why I haven't thought of Tosca before. The Castel Sant' Angelo where she threw herself off the walls is clearly visible from our terrace.

I hum a little from Mario's last aria and nod to a well-dressed stranger who seems to want to share my table. His name is Emilio Sacchetti and he wants to talk. This is unusual for strangers in Rome unless they are adolescents on the make. He starts by complaining that he is only a duke, he'd rather be a prince. In any case there are too many people in Rome who have his rank, mostly Germans. It infuriates him. His grandparents are buried in the church across from us and his father lives in the Sacchetti Palace. He should be the heir but his father has married a young and beautiful woman who has usurped his place. I cluck sympathetically. People think Rome is so romantic, but history can weigh heavy. It isn't all coronets and ermine. People's ideas of what is important changes—even the church has shrunk in importance just in my lifetime.

Hannah hates pretentious people. When she comes back with her melons she exchanges a few words with the duke and immediately dislikes him. He looks like a complainer, she says later. In Auschwitz the privileged were often the first to die. Unable to do anything for themselves, they would fall into a state of shock when they were treated just like everybody else. She takes my arm and we saunter back across the Corso to straighten up a bit before our friends arrive.

I see why Hannah wanted to have Stefano over. Arianne had been complaining that he was depressed. Not even their daughter's new baby girl could cheer him up. Oh I know, I know; I think I called him something else when I mentioned him before. If I did that's not because of my memory issues. It's because Hannah and Arianne are friends. Arianne confides in Hannah. She would feel dreadful to see his name in print. I planned to erase it later, though of course I might forget.

Luckily it was a beautiful day and we sat outside under a Titian blue sky filled with puffy white clouds while Arianne complained about Israel's settlement policy and threats to bomb Iran. She comes from a famous Jewish merchant family and gets as angry at Israel as if it were her own wayward child.

"It's crazy. They're suicidal," she said. Hannah agrees with her.

Stefano just shook his head. Arianne kept trying to interest him in the discussion but the medicine he is taking doesn't really seem to help him. It just makes him sleepy. I feel a sudden chill even though the day is warm. Am I looking at myself a year from now?

I've been reading more about Alzheimer's. They have been sending electrical stimulation to the portion of the brain where Auschwitz—what an odd mistake—I mean Alzheimer's, starts. The electric charge not only stops the disease from progressing—when given to mice, of course, creatures quite different from men—the stimulation also brings back the lost memory from 60 to 90 percent. The memory that improves is called spatial memory. The researchers tested it by a game of taxi where the goal is to drop off passengers at selected spots in an unfamiliar city.

Something snaps into place in my head. I have a faulty navigational system. It's not disease. I've had it as long as I can remember. Here in Rome, no matter how often I walk Governo Vecchio to Piazza Navona, I can't remember where a certain shop is. Or the gym where I used to work out three times a week. In the same way, across the Corso I don't remember the stores on Banchi Vecchi, in particular the one where I have many times bought dresses for Hannah.

Stefano is half asleep, his eyelids heavy. He opens his eyes and looks at me. I try to think of something amusing and tell him the joke about three Texans in a bar boasting about how much property they own. The first two talk about their tens of thousands of acres, King Ranch, Hot Springs Valley. The smallest man says he owns ten acres and they look at him amazed at his poverty. "What do you call it?" they ask. "Oh," he says, "Downtown Dallas." Stefano gives me the hint of a smile. He looks defeated. It's too hard to struggle. There was a group in the death camps that had given up hope of returning to normal life, of returning to any life. They were called "*Mussulmen*" and strenuously avoided. I understood. Without thinking, I moved my chair subtly away from him, though he's not in such dire straits and even if he were.... Under the table Arianne reached out and took Stefano's hand, squeezing it. Helping him hang on to life.

I was depressed after their visit and decided to get a massage to waken my flesh. I have a masseuse, a sweet young woman. She came around four o'clock with her lotions and her folding massage table. I lie with my privates covered by a towel and watch her jiggling breasts. They're not so big but the curve of them as they rise into her blouse is delicious, enchanting. As she bends over me, her hands lightly oiled, and starts to work on my shoulders and arms, I have to force myself to look away, picking a spot next to her left ear so as not to be rude.

"My shoulder is still causing me trouble," I tell her, "and my hip too. The right one. Probably from sitting at the computer."

She says we'll get to that later. She starts telling me about her trouble with a teenage daughter. I barely listen, responding with the obligatory "Uh huh" or "that must be hard." Meanwhile something else is getting hard, luckily hidden beneath the towel. I'd like to boast about it to her—at my age and all that. It feels so spritely. But I imagine she wouldn't be pleased. Once in Florence I was teaching a film course at the university, which incidentally has a fine psychology department. While I was in residence I went to a lecture on *perfezionismo* by a famous doctor—I'm not sure why, maybe I just loved the word—the desire to make perfect, to be perfect. Don't I have a bit of that, or was it just the desire to be right, which is quite a different thing?

Anyway, this gorgeous girl always sat in the front row mesmerizing the professor as her breasts rose and fell with her breath and she looked at him doe-eyed, drinking in the wisdom flowing from his parted lips. On the last day of the semester she came to his office and thanked him for being the first male in her life who seemed to be able to see beyond her tits.

My masseuse asks me to turn over, which I do briskly, taking care to hide my erection. She starts to knead my buttocks strongly. I point to the spot that hurts and she tells me that two muscles meet there. She presses so hard it hurts. I am conscious of how close she is to my anus. I imagine her reaching between my extended legs and massaging my balls very gently. Despite my excitement my erection is faltering. Fantasy can take me only so far.

Before I know it she is finishing up. I make another appointment for next week.

There was an article in the paper today about the Holocaust memorial in Israel, Yad Vashem. It has grown into a huge museum with audio tours in fifty languages. There is an accompanying photo of a group of serious-faced Asians looking at an exhibit. I wonder if they were comparing what they saw in it with what their grandparents may have suffered. At Hiroshima.

It's odd, having lived with Hannah all these years, that I never saw Lanzmann's famous film, *Shoah*. But maybe I didn't need to. I lived with it. The last survivors, like Hannah, are dying out. What will happen then? What will happen in this new century? Will the memories get fainter and fainter as they pass to the children of survivors and then to the grand-children?

We know several children of survivors, some very neurotic, others less so. Most are struggling with anxiety and fear. Some project it forward onto their children. I look at the photo of the Asian women. One of them said that she was afraid she would be depressed but that she had found the audio commentary unexpectedly inspiring because of the way the prisoners helped each other. Primo Levi wouldn't have agreed. He said the prisoners had one aim—to preserve and consolidate their privileges vis-a-vis the weaker ones. Isn't this what is happening today in our country? The rich grind down the poor who are in turn indignant that the poorest among them may get something they don't deserve. Hypocrisy flourishes along with religion.

When my eyes tire, I listen to *Slumdog Millionaire*, the novel that was made into a film that won an Oscar. The author compares the slum dwellers, the garbage collectors, to the prisoners of the camps—they too try continually to consolidate their position vis–a–vis the poorest of the poor. She follows the life of one of them who arouses envy in his fellows, who in revenge accuse him of a crime he didn't commit, ruining him, perhaps sending him to jail for life.

Primo, though I didn't know him well, was an admirable man. He pointedly tells how when he found a pipe leaking water, he shared it with his best friend but not with a third because the water might not have been enough for three. The story is a beautiful mix of generosity and calculation of what was necessary to survive. Still, Primo, seeing his dehydrated third friend feverish, dragging himself along with caked dried lips, felt ashamed and questioned the morality of what he'd done. Eventually his friend discovered traces of water on the pipe. Afterward when they had both survived, their friendship was never the same. My own feeling is that for each who shared a last piece of bread, there were many who refused to share, even if they themselves had enough. Human nature may be worse than we think.

I am depressed. If I weren't, I'd remember that there are plenty of examples in Primo's books of people who helped him at considerable risk, like the German who left him extra food every day at the fence where they were working. Or the illiterate man—I can't remember if he was a guard or a prisoner—who copied out Primo's letter to his mother and sent it. Hannah—saying I tend to remember the bad things and forget the good—would remind me of the guard in Auschwitz who let her lick his plate, always leaving some small scrap. She wasn't formally religious but for her, he was God!

Thinking about human nature, I am reminded of a rather sick game called Who Will Hide Me?" I don't remember exactly how it was played, but the question was which of a player's friends would betray him and which would hide him. I wondered what I would do. I was fairly sure I wouldn't inform on anyone, but to risk my neck to hide someone was another story. Right away I hear myself protesting that there is no hiding place either here or in Todi. The outbuildings have no cellars or attics. Then too there is my age—though you would think that being nearly finished would make me more willing to help. It embarrasses me that despite my years of conscious effort, I still often feel like a victim.

My mother, brought up in luxury, always portrayed herself as a victim struggling to stay alive, endlessly complaining that her own mother neglected her and moaning that if it rained and she wet her feet, she might die. But you don't drown in a rainstorm, even without an umbrella.

At this point I think I have to say that I'm distorting the facts. I said I found my mother unconscious. I think I remember feeling a lot of pain and then I remember feeling nothing, not even wanting to cry at her funeral. I was angry; very, very angry. So angry that I killed her off. That's right, she didn't really die when I was eight, she lived (the way Primo's mother did) to cause me years of pain. She lived as you might expect someone who had been an inmate of the camps to live—in constant fear. As if she had suffered horribly. I amplified every danger just the way she did. Rain, minor illness, staying up too late—everything. And like her I tried to justify doing that. I kept wanting to compare myself to other victims: wasn't I in some way a survivor even though not physically harmed, starved, or beaten? Maybe if I had strap marks, bruises, scars people would—would what? Love me, pity me. Now I can almost laugh about it. I still have my regressive moments. Like Phillip Roth lying on his analyst's couch complaining, transformed into the breast he wants to suckle.

I'm not sure exactly how it happened but as I began to have some success with my films, I became less and less a wallower. Subtly I flipped into being the one who takes care. Hannah gave me a great opportunity to do that. Caring for her all those years, I was a real mensch, or I like to think I was.

But I fell down. I was a schmuck, I made life difficult for the one person I loved most. I didn't make Claudia happy either. But when Hannah had her heart attack, I thought of it as a second chance to be caring. I asked her to let me come back home. She did, she let me. She was afraid of having another attack. I went with her everywhere, and I think she liked it. Then, ironically, I began to have trouble with my memory.

Now instead of my caring for Hannah she is caring for me. She does it with kindness but also wry humor and sometimes a glint of something else—a sense of her own power. Like anyone else she can get tired and cross.

My journey home started when I was visiting Hannah at the apartment after her heart attack, when she told me she was afraid of going too far from home and the nearby hospital. She told me that her doctor wanted her to have one of those devices where all you have to do is press a button and you get help.

"But what if I can't press it? What if I pass out?" she wondered.

"Maybe you should have someone here with you," I ventured.

"I couldn't stand to have some stranger wandering around while I'm working. There aren't any doors to close. It was hard enough for me when you were with me," she paused. "But then you had your own writing to keep you busy and you used to work outside on the terrace when the weather was good."

"I could do it again," I said. "I still like the terrace. If I'm not working, I could feed the gulls, water the plants. You might think of me as an extra pair of hands."

"Don't be silly, it would make you frightfully nervous to be looking out for me all the time, noticing if I looked pale in the morning, freezing like a pointer dog if I put my hand to my chest, if I cough. Scolding me when I forget my pills. If you felt suffocated before—that was what you said, wasn't it? Suffocated? You must have been with Claudia already. I sensed something. I thought that if I cosseted you enough, pampered you, you'd turn back to me. But you only felt more constrained."

That's exactly how it had been. She made a quiet nest for me, gave me everything she could.

"I'd promise not to fuss," I said. "I'd just be there when you need me." She smiled with her mouth but her eyes were doubtful.

"You really want to come back," she asked, "for me?"

"For both of us, if you could forgive me. Do you think you could?"

Then a few days later she visited me. "Do you still want to come back?" she asked me. "I thought it wouldn't be right to take advantage of a moment of weakness."

For answer I kissed her.

It's probably understandable that I tried to minimize the importance of my time with Claudia. I hated to admit to myself that Hannah probably guessed I was having an affair long before I moved out. During that time she was more afraid than ever of being alone. I travelled a lot but I always called her and wrote to her even when it was only a short trip.

Dearest Hannle hannah panna my love, I miss you, kiss you. The endearments multiplied as I tried to tug free.

After, I moved out, you can imagine how painful that was. It was spring when I left and she insisted on keeping my winter clothes, my wool trousers, my heavier jackets, in a closet.

"Maybe you'll be back by winter," she said. "We'll be together again."

Later she confessed that she would go into that closet regularly to smell and caress my things. She kept other things too: ornaments and mementos from our trips. I didn't want her to feel any more bereft than she had to. I didn't want the apartment—formerly ours—to seem empty. She kept the paintings and most of the books. I would come in sometimes and see her dusting them with a big feather duster. And I left her almost all the Limoges plates, and pots from the little kitchen. I kept only what was absolutely necessary. (Claudia was less restrained and had taken with her a generous half of her menage with the dentist.)

Hannah's sister and niece, Leah and Sarah, came to visit during the early months of our separation. Leah was horrified to find that we weren't living together. Like a child with estranged parents, she kept trying to draw me back into the family circle. She was sure Hannah had done something to "lose" me. Hannah hadn't told her about our parting, guessing that her sister wouldn't understand.

I didn't want Hannah to be embarrassed or harassed and I visited, took them out to dinner, acted normally insofar as I could and kept deflecting Leah's questions.

"You look as if you're at the dentist's and want to jump out of the chair as soon as you can," Leah said.

The irony was unintended. I couldn't help smiling. Hannah's sister couldn't figure it out. I did my best, talked about needing space for awhile, having an important project to finish. Would it have been better to stay away from them? Maybe.

I guess I was trying to show Hannah that living this way was an option. It was possible. She could enjoy her freedom and enjoy seeing me too. I celebrated holidays with her, brought her presents, took her out to dinner, called regularly to check on her. But she was so sensitive. If my tone was slightly preoccupied, if I weren't engaging with her completely, she felt tortured. But how about me? Do you think it was easy for me to see her distress? Now I had to accept that she wanted to give our script a happy ending, even if it arrived only in old age, two ancient people living together again, surrounded by flowers. And here we are.

But where did all that pain go? Back then I often felt how hard it was for her to accept my invitations graciously, though what she really wanted to do was scream at me, plead with me, dramatize her eternal love.

If, for instance, I asked her to out with me on New Year's and then told her I'd be away for Christmas—shorthand for being with Claudia—she would have to keep tight control and not complain or withdraw. I knew that, but I still wanted what I was doing to be out in the open. Was that so wrong? She would withdraw into a hard shell, like a tortoise. Conversation would slow and stop. Eventually I would take her back to what was now her place as if she were a tired child and put her to bed, where, she told me, she would lie awake for hours staring at the ceiling.

There was an article in the *International Herald Tribune* today on drugs that cloud your mind. I used to like to read several papers, *Figaro*, the *Corriere della Sera*. Now it is just the *Tribune* because it is short and easy to get through. I think this was the second time they published an article on fuzzy brains. Apparently if you take both a calcium channel breaker, which I do because of a single event of heart spasm, and a statin, the combination can turn you into a zombie. The codeine cough syrup the doctor prescribed to keep me from moving around in my sleep can apparently have a similar effect. So which do I chose—a broken head or a fuzzy brain? You'd think it would be a cinch to decide—go for clearing the brain, I mean. But I'm afraid of seriously injuring myself if I throw myself out of bed. I could hit the radiator.

If I'm adding up the pros and cons, I should mention that I dropped my pill organizer on the floor in the bathroom and had trouble getting the pills back in the right order.

"You're just not concentrating," Hannah says.

Then she is sorry at sounding harsh and offers to go out for a walk with me. We walk in the sunshine over to San Luigi dei Francesi and look at the marvelous Caravaggios, which perfectly fit my mood. Wasn't Christ the supreme altruist? As usual I puzzle over Saint Matthew being chosen by Christ standing ghost-like in the doorway of the room where the men are playing cards. Matthew points to his chest, incredulous at being the chosen one. After you look at it awhile it seems almost as if he is pointing to the man next to him, saying, no, not me, him. No, that's not Matthew; it's what I would do. Matthew grew into the job.

The illumination kept going off. Italians are stingy that way, often leaving it to someone else to put in a coin. Finally, a dapper little man with a goatee, after looking scornfully around him at the crowd pressing against the railing, dropped in a coin. And the lights blazed up. Hannah and I smiled at each other, holding little fingers, and for a moment felt like new lovers, still lovers after all this time.

When we got home I saw that I had misplaced my reading glasses. I had used them in the church to see the details close up. I was sure I had asked Hannah to put them back in her purse; she had been carrying them for me just so they wouldn't get lost. We lapsed into a chorus of recriminations. The mood is broken.

It seems as if every hour I do something which irritates Hannah. I keep track of the days and my plans on my BlackBerry—gift from Hannah, of course. I never was very good at keeping my plans straight and now I'm worse. I can't tell if it is age or a brain filled with plaque, the debris of a lifetime of thinking, gradually returning a man to his animal state, but without the easy pleasure or the knowledge of how to hunt and kill. Even balance and ease of gait, lost. See, I tell myself, I can think well enough. But would I notice if I couldn't?

It's better not to think about that too much. In any case right now I am on a plateau. The doctor agrees, and this journal certainly helps me hold on to what I've been and done, to who I am.

I had a long talk with Erminia, our *donna di servizio* who comes twice a week to clean and wash. I found myself wishing she came more often. She is almost a member of the family. But she still works on her own family's farm, sows and reaps, takes care of the animals. And when she's too old to do that, there are her grandchildren. It would be good to be one of them, I think. She never finds fault and is resolutely cheerful, always telling me how well I look, how handsome, a little as if I were a child, patting my cheek.

I follow her as she waters, the way I used to tag after my wet nurse, a woman I imagine or partially remember, generously built, solid on her two legs, able to pick up fifty kilos of grain, to work all day in a good humor, carrying me in a pack on her back, talking to herself and me about the olive crop. Erminia's two sons don't know how to work the land, she tells me sadly. My mother, in a gesture from another age, put me with a wet nurse until I was three or four and this gave me whatever sense I have of easy-going, loving family life.

Hannah never wanted to have a room of her own. No that's not true. She never liked sleeping with all her sisters and brothers in one bed, didn't like the noises coming from behind the curtain where her parents slept. And here our *attico* has just one room, one space where you can shut the door. She insisted that I take it. She could work in the living room or, when it was nice, out on the terrace. I took the library, as we call it, without much thought and now am stuck here, impotent, surrounded by shelves of books while she clacks away.

She never used to write so steadily but it's her new project, the one she is doing about the daughter of a Holocaust survivor whose husband, a Catholic, is unfaithful with a Palestinian woman. She says it is about the possibility of peace between the three great faiths. A friend to whom she showed her manuscript said she thought Hannah hated the Palestinian woman and was prejudiced, but Hannah swore that wasn't true. She wants to know the woman and forgive.

I wonder then if it is about us. The Jewish wife has a mother who had survived the camps and is terribly anxious about everything. Maybe Hannah has found the perfect plot to embody our story, except that she is the survivor, not her mother, and Claudia is a Catholic only on holidays.

I can't say it isn't an interesting idea to show how her characters' beliefs affect their love affairs. It is! But if her work obsesses her, consumes her, I can feel it only as a rival. Or as if I am dead already and she is going on with her life with renewed vigor. I said that to her—one of those things you know you shouldn't say but say anyway.

"You are healthy as a horse," she said. "I'm the one likely to die. You don't have to talk like that to get my sympathy," she kisses me on the brow. Being able to take the high ground always pleases her. She goes downstairs and comes back after a few minutes with a hot chocolate and a *cornetto*.

"I'm not myself this morning," I say. "I'm sorry."

"It's nothing," she lies. But it isn't nothing. It's how things are now. Things trigger me, set me off. Anxiety like a dirty fog condenses into something harsher, hysterical—chokes me.

"Please don't leave me," I murmur so low that she doesn't hear.

It's Easter. The bells ring out from all the churches. When I was small we used to hide eggs in the garden after my mother and I had decorated them, dipping them in crimson and blue, my favorite colors. She was good at things like this, my mother. Things like egg painting or taffy pulling that had no hint of the practical.

Hannah, with no memories of the Christian holiday, is working away in the living room. Suddenly I hear her push back her chair and close her typewriter. "I'm going for a walk," she calls to me. I don't suggest going with her because the weather is grim. Every few minutes the sky spits rain on the terrace, then abruptly pours down, flooding the gutters, licking at the glass door. I crawl back into the new bed where I lie safely next to the wall and fiddle with myself, lazily watching the seagulls circling, trying to hold their course in the wind. The wind whips the white wisteria that Hannah planted, which is blossoming for the first time. If it keeps on like this there will be no more blossoms left by nightfall. A cold draft comes through the partly opened door.

Why isn't Hannah here to comfort me? She says walking in the wind and rain scours her brain, giving it a fresh space for ideas. She's gotten to the dead center of the new book. Now there is no question of changing course. She's waited so long for this. When she first came here and spoke up for the Palestinians, people refused to listen. Who was it who spoke of literature as sugarcoating a bitter pill? Someone in the seventeenth century? That's what she's doing now, hiding the medicine. I can tell she isn't quite satisfied, though she doesn't complain. I'm sure it's good but she always wants more. Sometimes when she is reading one of the classics, Dante, Primo Levi, Calvino, I walk into the living room and find her crying because she can never be great.

Last night we watched the pope's Easter procession at the Coliseum on television. He looked like an impotent old man, hands clasped in prayer, one finger pointing upward, dressed in his gorgeous clothes, high above the thousands trying to get a glimpse of him. Maybe he was thanking God for holding back the thunderstorm, due yesterday. The clergy is in enough trouble. God, your church is besieged on all sides. Maybe he promises more mortification of his flesh. Pronounces himself a willing victim and wishes for a miracle to revive the ancient roots. Looking out over the crowd, I thought the only people who looked genuine were the African nuns.

Hannah came back from her walk exultant and announced that she was going to take a break and go back with me to visit my family's old place, our tower near Todi in Torre Gentile. I think I mentioned it before—we had gone for the weekend and Hannah wouldn't let me drink wine. I haven't done or said anything provocative this morning but it is so easy to make her feel guilty, just by a turn of my head or a hint of dullness in my voice. I'm sure she wants me to see how much she cares for me by interrupting her work just when it is going well, trying to make up for being so immersed in it. But why shouldn't she be? Didn't I do the same thing for years? Of course I did. And I didn't just work at home; even before our separation I traveled regularly to conferences and festivals. She always hated my trips, suspecting that I was having a fling. Even if I did it meant nothing.

It's funny how just thinking of the time when I was the prime mover, so to speak, makes me feel stronger, clearer in my mind, but also makes me want to blame Hannah for my mental troubles. I catch myself doing that and give myself a mental slap.

"I'm packing a picnic," Hannah says from the doorway.

"It's a lovely idea but..." I gesture at the rain-streaked door.

"The rain is supposed to stop in an hour or so," she says, "and if it doesn't we can start a fire when we get there." There are two huge fireplaces, one upstairs in the bedroom, the other down in the rustic kitchen, and a fine pile of cut wood near each of them. When the fire is lit there is always a musky smell.

My heart always beats harder when I get near Torre Gentile, passing through the beautiful valley with its gray olive trees—most of them replanted by the government after the exodus from the farms. The fields are a mass of yellow mustard flowers and there is an orange moss on the next door roof. The colors modulate nicely—an impressionist's dream. The house itself is gray stone with a massive base from the time when it still had its tower, first line of defense for the little town. Slits cut in the walls for the archers to shoot from are now widened and filled with glass, and a big glass window has been cut into the stone facing the fields of olive trees.

I know that it was built in the fourteen hundreds, but I can't recall when it lost its tower and became our summer home.

Hannah was right. The rain became a fine mist and we lay on fur rugs in front of the fire and looked at the flames or up at the huge beams. I used to cut the logs myself, but now our custodian does it and there are firesticks to make it catch.

We hear doves cooing in the trees. Hannah puts her arms around me and hugs me tight. Then she unpacks the picnic basket. The food—*foie gras*, my favorite cheeses, fresh bread, peaches—and Hannah's warmth carries away my angry thoughts. When the fire sinks down, she puts on a fresh log, spreads pâté on the bread for me, tucks a napkin under my chin—these days I tend to dribble a little—caring for me the way I used to for her. Why do we have to grow old? Each day losing more ground, walking less far, limbs shaky, slipping and sliding, losing the very qualities that made us attractive. I'm beginning to see why some people kill themselves to avoid this.

May 1, the day when the workers of Italy celebrate. We are back in town. The stores will be closed all day, some longer because of other holidays added on. I can't believe I used to be moved by the tricolor, the planes swooping by, leaving behind a trail of red, white and green. I could see it all from the terrace, vibrant against the blue of the sky. Now the Italian Left is no better than anyone else, almost as lifeless as the American. I think of poor Lucian, exiled to Mexico for ten years, cutting wood with George. All the time sustained by his belief in father Stalin.

The last time I saw him alive his wife was saying, "We've lived too long." They outlived both their bodies and their friends. Poor Gabriella. She got terribly depressed. But at least she could still get out with help. Lucian was reduced to a crawl, using the walker as extra legs, that plastic bag clearly visible inside his robe, having to work so hard just to keep himself together—pulling the tie of his purple robe closed was just too much to ask.

"I'm going to pieces," he said, "my hearing, my eyes."

I thought then that they had made a bargain. He had the physical pain, she the mental. Lucian fought off his own depression by living in his memories. You just had to mention the blacklist, and he'd be off telling his story of how when he had come back from Mexico he was hired under a false name by Harry Cohn the head of Columbia Pictures. Cohn was the only one in Hollywood who met him in person, everyone else insisted on not seeing him, so if they were investigated they could say they didn't know him. Cohn kept Kim Novak as a sex slave, and she used to crawl under his desk and give him blow jobs. Lucian and a pal worked for a whole year on the film with the actors and a whole crew, but then Columbia dropped it. No one wanted to get in trouble.

It didn't matter how many times Lucian had told this story, it always brought a faint glow to his cheeks and brightened his eyes. Rita Hayworth was Cohn's star too but she wouldn't sleep with him.

"Keep it in your pants, Harry," she famously said. "I'm having lunch with your wife tomorrow." And here Lucian always laughed.

Nietzsche used to say that memory was overrated: one should live in the present. That would be good if I could do it without anger! Personally, I like the Jungian idea of a world soul, a flowing together of memories. Already I see that happening, my memories merging with Hannah's, my brother's, Lucian's. When one dies the others carry on. That's probably why people are so determined to have children. To carry on. There is a nugget of truth in memories and maybe it won't matter who experienced them first. No best or final. I picture it as a warm cloud filled with images, very beautiful.

But doesn't this flowing together of memories go against the historians who are always trying to dig out details of the past? And didn't someone say the individual is always struggling not to be overwhelmed by the tribe? I am soothed by the collective soul flowering tangibly in the great cathedrals of the Middle Ages. No one pointed to a particularly expressive figure with his pants down or a devil with a long penis and admitted, "Those things are mine." No, they are ours, our sinful thoughts.

It strikes me like an ache in my chest how much I still want recognition, praise. I go out on the terrace and wait for the lift in my spirits when I step into the dappled sunshine cast by the leaves of a blooming tree whose name escapes me. I let it go. The delicate flowers are reflected in the glass tabletop along with the dark green pine, its base surrounded by fragments of Roman sculpture, a present from an archaeologist friend. The variety of greens and tender flowering plants soothes like a salve. I walk to the edge and look for the young gulls. There are three, one more than last year. I notice for the first time that the parent who is sitting placidly to one side, has black-and-white tail feathers. I hear the chicks squeaking plaintively for food, but they'll have to wait until their foraging parent comes back. One looks distinctly weaker and I wonder if he'll die.

After a few minutes the parent returns and the little ones peck frantically at her beak until she releases the food. I notice with relief that even the weaker one gets something. When their parent moves away, they follow her, stumbling over the red tiles, up the red side and down into the browner trough that matches their feathers. She leads them like a Pied Piper down to the very edge of the roof. Is she considering leading them like lemmings into the void? Is she already tired of mothering? You see, I assume she is female. The weaker chick takes a few steps inside the nest, lacking the courage to hasten after his siblings. The mother pauses a moment to see if the shaky one will join them. She stands right on the edge with the others. I worry that a strong gust of wind could blow the chicks down. My attention is riveted. I feel totally involved in what could be the survival of the fittest.

Hannah comes to the terrace door and asks if I had done the stretches the physical therapist had recommended for my hip. Yes, I said, annoyed to be reminded of my body. It was true I had done them, desultorily. I look away from her. She can always read my expression and see that I am lying by a slight wrinkle in my forehead or fear in my eyes that change their color from blue to gray. My *bocca della verita*, I call her, after the big stone sculpture of an open-mouthed river god who bites the fingers of liars.

I look furtively into the terrace next door to see if my little boy is there, but he isn't. I notice that I'm coming to think of him as mine, realizing how much I miss not having a grandchild, someone with my genes. Hannah sighs and looks for a moment as if she is going to tell me something important; but she only sighs again and goes back to her desk. I give her a few minutes and then go inside. I walk casually to the bathroom and on the way back go over and kiss her on the neck.

She is staring at something that she covers hastily but not before I see the letter announcing that she has won a prestigious prize. She has leaned the announcement against a photo so she can see it better. The photo is of me. "Lifetime achievement award," she says smiling up at me. She waits for a response.

"You deserve it," I say, nuzzling her neck.

As though she senses the grudging nature of my acknowledgment, she moves away.

"I have to write a letter now sweetheart, then I'll go and get us something nice for lunch al fresco," she says. "I hope the elevator doesn't act up. The *signora* next door told me it had gone dead twice. She told me that I should wait until I hear the door click before pressing the floor button."

I hardly listen. The main point that enters my awareness is that she is going out soon. It strikes me that I'd feel better if she were depressed. Her cheerfulness makes me more unhappy. She takes my ailments in stride, as long as she has that old typewriter of hers and can pound away on it.

I walk back to the terrace, feeling like an old lion pacing in its cage. How can I feel so ungenerous towards Hannah when I spent years building her up, showing her how to make use of the terrible things that happened to her, turn them into art? And now that she has succeeded, how can I begrudge this, especially as she continues to acknowledge what I gave her? And she seems almost glad of my weaknesses so she can show her willingness to care. I shake myself. Stop it! I go out to the terrace and sit with eyes closed, listening to the sound of my little wall fountain. It makes the space magical, a fourth dimension away from any care. I can imagine being beside a gentle brook—the kind that sings over small stones, and bubbles. There was a brook like that at the edge of our vineyards up in Todi. It came from a deep spring and I used to go "fishing" there with a string on a stick. I can't remember catching anything. Probably there were no fish, though the word *catfish* keeps coming to my mind.

While I am refreshing myself with memories of the deep green of the trees surrounding the spring, I hear Roberto saying hello. He is on the other side of the lattice, of course, and he says *ciao* so softly that it could almost be the voice of my fountain, but when I open my eyes there he is.

"Would you like to come and visit?" I ask.

"Yes," he says, "I would."

So I get the key off the top of my *armàdio* just inside the door and I open the lattice. The *signora* had put out the wash earlier, and the shirts and jeans and underwear are waving in the breeze. She must have hung them very quietly. I wasn't aware of her doing it.

"I see you didn't bring your book," I say. "Would you like to have more *Oz*? I'd be glad to read to you."

He looks down at his feet.

"Mama took my book for the day as a punishment for teasing the baby."

"What were you doing?" I ask him.

"I was only playing," he answers. "I'd put out a finger and he'd try to catch it."

"Maybe he's a little young for that," I said.

"He tried but he couldn't—then he started to cry. If she had left us alone I would have let him…" He paused, looking unhappy.

"I'm sure you would have," I said, somewhat insincerely, remembering my brother's taunts and petty cruelties.

"I'd like to go out," he said all of a sudden, "and get an ice cream. You know, downstairs to the bar."

They had a particularly nice selection—all homemade with pure natural ingredients. Before I could think of any reason not to undertake this adventure, I took him by the hand. What better way to soothe an unhappy child? Eating ice cream was one of the best memories of my childhood—the mouth still longing for the breast, placated by the cool semiliquid, the licking and sucking.

"What a good idea," I said looking down at him. The *signora* might not like it—my mind skittered away from her possible disapproval—but we could be there and back in a jiffy.

No reason why she had to know.

A few minutes later Roberto and I stood in front of the trays, drinking in the sight of the mounds: raspberry and mixed fruit, chocolate truffle, chocolate with orange, chocolate chip, cookies and cream, sorbets in bright colors.

"Maybe I should bring some back for Mama," he said, "and the baby." His handsome face took on a worried expression as though he was trying to work out a puzzle that was too hard for his age.

"Let's have ours first," I said. "Then we'll think about what to get them." He shuffled from foot to foot. "In fact it might be better if we kept our little outing a secret between us two."

"I wish you had a magic spell to make us invisible or a belt like Dorothy's that could zip us home in a flash."

"Don't worry," I said. "We'll take some back with us. Just relax now and enjoy your cone. You'd better lick around the other side. It's going to drip." I stopped short of saying, "you'll really make Mama mad." What was the matter with me? My thoughts kept turning to times when I'd had the best intentions but things turned out badly, like making a birthday cake for my mother and putting in salt instead of sugar. I shouldn't have even been in the kitchen and the cook, one of the few servants I really liked, got fired.

"Pick two flavors for them. Don't worry. I'll explain."

He looked dubious. We took wild berry and chocolate and I carried the bag for him while he licked slowly around his cone's volcanic tip.

Our elevator is uncertain in the best of times, a green metal box with faux-wood trim. As we got in I tried to remember what Hannah had said about its newest glitch, something about waiting, but it seemed to be working all right. Roberto was dancing from one foot to another. Either he was excited at the thought of giving ice cream to his new Mama or he had to pee. The elevator crawled slowly up to the fifth floor and stopped. Roberto threw open the inner door. Too late. I remembered we should have waited to hear a click as the mechanism released. I felt a chill, my hand trembled as I tried the door myself. It wouldn't open. Roberto looked stricken.

"Don't worry," I told him. "One of the neighbors will come by and I bet they can open the doors from the outside. While we wait maybe you could tell me what you were up to in *The Magic of Oz* book. Or more about how the characters from all the books come to you at night and you imagine adventures for them before you go to sleep."

"I was up to where Captain Bill nails the Beast to the ground with a stake. He doesn't die because nothing dies in Oz."

"But he can be kept from harming anyone."

"Yes," sighs Roberto.

I seem to remember being reassured as a child by the absence of death in the *Oz* stories—did I write about that before? It was clearly a comfort to Roberto. Who knows? He may even imagined going to find his dead parents. Though of course he may not have imagined anything of the kind.

Just then I heard the heavy front door bang shut and what sounded like our downstairs neighbor, a loud-voiced blond whose parents owned the *fruttivendolo* down the block, talking to her dog. Then I heard her cursing to herself, "*Porco madonna. Porco miseria,*" as she tried to get a response from the elevator, gave up, and slowly climbed up the stairs. When I thought she had gotten to her floor, I called out to her that we were stuck. Could she help? She climbed the extra floor with still more curses and tried our elevator door. No luck.

"Is there someone else who could help? A repair man?"

She pulled out her cell phone—I could see her though the grill—and called.

"He won't be back until tomorrow morning," she flipped her phone shut.

"What! We have to stay here overnight? That's impossible. I have a child here with me."

Roberto who had been listening intently, started to cry.

"I have to pee," he moaned, "I really have to pee."

Just then the blond's elderly mother appeared, with a second sausage-shaped dog on a leash. It was getting to be like a Becket play.

"Don't worry *poverino*, don't *piànge*. Poor little thing," she said. "You can pee through the grate."

Just then the sausage dog started to bark.

"Zitta, quiet," she yelled at him. "Your neighbor next door might have a wire," she said, "*Signora* Bussola. I'll ask her."

Signora Bussola was Roberto's new Mama. He moaned.

"The ice cream we got for her is melting," he sobbed. "It's coming right through the box."

"Here, I'll take it," I said. I took out my pocket handkerchief and made a show of wrapping it around the bottom of the container, though I knew it would soak through in a few minutes. Still, it quieted Roberto.

A more serious problem was that I was having to pee as well. It happened regularly whenever I got close to home. These days, usually by the time I got to the front door, there'd be a terrible urgency. I'd have to rush for the bathroom. I could feel the urgency growing as the blond's father joined the group outside the elevator. Then when I was thinking this couldn't get any worse, I saw a new pair of legs outside the grill, and I heard Roberto's new Mama's voice.

"What in the world is going on," she asked. "Roberto are you in there?" she barked. I wondered how I'd ever been entranced by her nurturing qualities—how nice she was with her baby.

"Yes," Roberto rubbed his nose with his sleeve. "And I have to pee."

"I'll get my wire," she said, and I could hear a collective sigh from outside. "Just hold on, Roberto." But it is already too late. I can see the pale lemon liquid trickling down his leg beneath his shorts. He crouches in a corner of the elevator and puts his hands over his head as though that would make him invisible. I know how he feels. My bladder is clamoring to let go. I know in a few minutes it will start to leak and then…

I hear someone say in the high pitched voice Italians use when something dramatic is going on, "Move, give the *signora* some space."

There is the chink chink of metal against metal while she inserts her wire. I was too distressed to see exactly how it worked. But the door opened.

The *signora* walked into the elevator and took Roberto by the arm, pulled him outside, all the while peppering me with questions.

"How could you take him out without checking with me?" she asked in that operatic voice. "What sort of way is that to behave? I was about to call the police." She shook Roberto's arm. "Did he hurt you?" she asked. Roberto wouldn't look at her, he just kept crying.

"I got you ice cream," he whimpered. She softened slightly.

"You're just a child," she said pulling the container out of my hand and throwing it into a plastic container the blond held out to her. "He's just a child but you, Renzo." It suddenly hit me that she might think I was a pervert.

"Excuse me," I said with as much dignity as I could, "but I have to…" I pushed my way through the onlookers to my door and unlocked it. All the time I was turning the double bolt she followed behind me, pulling at my jacket, trying to get a response from me. "Remember, I am your landlady as well as your neighbor. This is not a game. I don't want you to have anything more to do with my son."

I managed to pull the door shut after me. I couldn't make it to the bathroom so I dashed into the terrace and peed in the corner by the drain. As I peed, I could still hear their voices.

A new voice was added, and I recognized my Hannah. My god, what if the *signora* wanted to evict us? She owns half the building. The rest of us only rent. She definitely has the decisive voice around here. After I finished and shook myself off I leaned out the window so I could hear better.

"No," I heard the *signora* say. "No, I meant what I said. I don't want him having anything more to do with Roberto."

"Renzo wasn't doing anything bad," Hannah is saying, remembering perhaps how quickly her village neighbors had turned against her. "It must have frightened you dreadfully and I'm really sorry. He's fond of the boy. Roberto is lonely. He has suffered a terrible blow. It seems like a perfect match. A marriage made in heaven." I hear Hannah laughing, trying to make light.

"Nothing happened, thank God," Roberto's new mother persists. "But it could have. If Renzo got distracted and one of those motorcycles came speeding around the corner. I just can't treat it as a lark." I could see that she wasn't going to bend.

"I don't want to seem cruel," she went on in a softer voice, "but I shouldn't have to tell you about Renzo's lapses of attention. I've seen him wandering around like a lost soul, not knowing where he is. What if he had the boy with him? And then there is the alarm. It has gone off three times in the last month because he used the wrong code. The security of the whole building depends on that alarm. People are starting to ignore it," she proclaimed. "I'm sorry to say that I think Renzo is a danger not just to Roberto but to the other tenants and to himself." For a moment I recognize the *signora* with the baby and am confused about which she is: monster or caring parent. Both? It is too complicated for me right now.

I go into the bathroom to take a shower and calm myself down.

As soon as I step inside I see that I'm not alone and jump back in alarm. There is a tall slender man with bushy eyebrows staring out at me with green eyes.

"Who are you?" I lash out at him. "What do you think you're doing?" It occurs to me that he is an addict stealing our pills. I try to call out but my voice sounds as if it's coming out of a deep well and Hannah doesn't hear me. Then I notice that the intruder is wrinkled and stooped. No need to get help, I could probably push him over. "Who are you?" I asked again. He seems about to answer. His lips move but if he says anything, I don't hear him. I reach out and touch cold glass. The intruder is me.

Shaken, I retreat to the shower. I want it hard, like a waterfall plummeting down around me, hiding me inside, but as usual it only trickles, an old man's shower. I know I can't hide inside it forever, but at least for a few minutes I can stand there, water warm on my shoulders, and think about what I can say to Hannah. She doesn't come right away, so I get out and dry myself, glancing every few minutes at the horror in the mirror. Finally I hear a light knocking at the door.

"What's happening in here," she asks, cracking the door. "I thought I heard you call. Are you alright?"

I mumble a yes and she opens the door and comes in.

"I know you can't help it," she says coming close and rubbing my shoulders, "but you can stop trembling. You're safe now. Better here with me than outside." She tries a smile. "But we do have to think about our landlady problem. You know she's a very nervous woman."

"I hadn't really noticed," I muttered.

"Remember what a fuss she made about your watering the plants too much? She was sure the water would come through her ceiling and wanted to make us put in a whole drip system. Came over one night when her husband was away and there was a thunderstorm. But even if she weren't afraid of everything, having a new child arrive from one day to the next without any warning, being responsible for him and a new baby. Oh, what's the point?" She said suddenly.

"I'm sorry," I murmured low. "I should have asked her permission."

"She's our landlady," Hannah said, and I saw her hand shake. "Her family owns half the building; she could evict us!"

"I didn't think of that." Whether I could have thought of it hung in the air.

Hannah looked at me hard. "We need to have someone here with you. At least in the mornings when I am working or shopping. I can't work if I'm worrying about you or about losing the apartment"—she lowers her voice—"about losing my home. You must see that." She lit a cigarette. "Don't worry. I'll find someone suitable but you have to help. You can't harass them like you did that woman from Guatemala."

"I just asked her what she was doing here and told her politely there was nothing I needed."

Hannah's face puckers up as if she were going to cry.

"You weren't polite; you yelled at her—'Why are you here? Who are you? I don't know you.' You screamed when she tried to wash your hair and after a week she left."

"I don't want some strange woman picking out my clothes for me, dressing me. It's humiliating, seeing me naked, can't you understand?"

She doesn't want to answer me. Instead she goes on with her thoughts. "That's why I've been helping you myself, this year and last year too. But after I help you dress in clean clothes and comb your hair just so, the way you like it, then when I go in to work you ask me when I'll be finished. Isn't that so? And then you ask me for a coffee and just when I am catching the thread again, another coffee and then the bathroom."

Her voice softens.

"And you say I should spoil you, do you remember? You don't leave me alone for five minutes, and if I say wait, you don't care."

I hang my head. I do remember, but I pictured myself charming and suave the way I was when Hannah's French friend was visiting and I spoke French easily, drank wine with them, and joked. Afterwards I heard her friend whisper that I seemed fine, coherent, full of talk as usual.

"I remember," I say. "But I don't think my judgment is impaired. I just wanted to take the boy out for ice cream."

"We have to get someone new, at least someone to help get you up in the morning, shower, go for a walk…"

"I'm not a dog," I say, getting louder, "needing to be walked."

"There's no choice anymore. We have to have someone, can't you see? Roberto's mother said you needed to be somewhere else, somewhere where you'd be cared for. If we don't get you this kind of help and you're on your own, something else will happen and she'll throw us out."

""Why don't you just put me on an ice floe and let me starve?" I heard myself yelling, and I couldn't stop. I wanted to shake her. Thank God I didn't. I just started to cry, my image of myself crumbling. "I'm just so frightened," I said.

"I know, I know," she said, and put her arms around me.

"Will you send me away?" I asked her.

I started to cry. I wanted to kneel at her feet, kiss her feet. I slumped to the floor and held on to her legs. She snuffed out her cigarette and pulled me up.

"No I won't," she said. "Never…ever."

I looked deep into her eyes and decided, at least for now, to believe her.

The End

About the Author

B renda Webster was born in New York City, educated at
Swarthmore, Barnard, Columbia, and Berkeley, where
she earned her Ph.D. She is a novelist, freelance writer,
playwright, critic and translator who splits her time between
Berkeley and Rome. Webster has written two controversial
and oft-anthologized critical studies, *Yeats: A Psychoanalytic
Study* (Stanford) and *Blake's Prophetic Psychology* (Macmillan).
She has translated poetry from the Italian for *The Other Voice*
(Norton) and *The Penguin Book of Women Poets*. She is co-
editor of the journals of the abstract expressionist painter (and
Webster's mother) Ethel Schwabacher, *Hungry for Light: The
Journal of Ethel Schwabacher* (Indiana 1993). She is the author
of four previous novels, *Sins of the Mothers* (Baskerville 1993),
Paradise Farm (SUNY, 1999), *The Beheading Game* (Wings
Press, 2006), which was a finalist for the Northern California
Book Award, and *Vienna Triangle* (Wings Press, 2009). Her
memoir, *The Last Good Freudian* (Holmes and Meier, 2000)
received considerable critical praise. The Modern Language
Association published Webster's translation of Edith Bruck's
Holocaust novel, *Lettera alla Madre,* in 2007. Webster's novel,
Vienna Triangle, "navigates between the late Sixties and *fin
de siecle* Vienna in a dramatic exploration of family romances
inside and outside the circle that so famously gathered
around the father of psychoanalysis, Sigmund Freud" (Sandra
Gilbert). Her new play, "The Murder Trial of Sigmund Freud,"
was inspired by *Vienna Triangle,* but goes beyond the story
of Tausk and Freud to chronicle Freud's relationships with
women patients, disciples and his family. "The Murder Trial
of Sigmund Freud" was written in collaboration with Meridee
Stein, who conceived the idea of a play and brought to the
table many stimulating ideas and twenty years of experience in
the theater. Webster is the president of PEN West.

Wings Press was founded in 1975 by Joanie Whitebird and Joseph F. Lomax, both deceased, as "an informal association of artists and cultural mythologists dedicated to the preservation of the literature of the nation of Texas." Publisher, editor and designer since 1995, Bryce Milligan is honored to carry on and expand that mission to include the finest in American writing—meaning all of the Americas, without commercial considerations clouding the choice to publish or not to publish.

Wings Press produces multicultural books, chapbooks, ebooks, CDs, and broadsides that, we hope, enlighten the human spirit and enliven the mind. Everyone ever associated with Wings has been or is a writer, and we believe that writing is a transformational art form capable of changing the world, primarily by allowing us to glimpse something of each other's souls. Good writing is innovative, insightful, open-minded, and interesting. But most of all it is honest.

Likewise, Wings Press is committed to treating the planet itself as a partner. Thus the press uses as much recycled material as possible, from the paper on which the books are printed to the boxes in which they are shipped.

As Robert Dana wrote in *Against the Grain,* "Small press publishing is personal publishing. In essence, it's a matter of personal vision, personal taste and courage, and personal friendships." Welcome to our world.

Colophon

This first edition of *After Auschwitz: A Love Story*, by Brenda Webster, has been printed on 55pound EB "natural" paper containing a percentage of recycled fiber. Titles have been set in Papyrus type, the text is in Adobe Caslon type. All Wings Press books are designed and produced by Bryce Milligan, publisher and editor.

On-line catalogue and ordering available at
www.wingspress.com

Wings Press titles are distributed
to the trade by the
Independent Publishers Group
www.ipgbook.com
and in Europe by
www.gazellebookservices.co.uk

Also available as an ebook.